The
ANTIDEPRESSANT
FACT BOOK

Books By Peter R. Breggin, M.D.

Nonfiction

College Students in a Mental Hospital: An Account of Organized
Social Contacts Between College Volunteers and Mental Patients in a
Hospital Community (1962) (Jointly authored with Umbarger et al.)

Electroshock: Its Brain-Disabling Effects (1979)

The Psychology of Freedom: Liberty and Love as a Way of Life (1980)

Psychiatric Drugs: Hazards to the Brain (1983)

Toxic Psychiatry: Why Therapy, Empathy and Love
Must Replace the Drugs, Electroshock and
Biochemical Theories of the "New Psychiatry" (1991)

Beyond Conflict: From Self-Help and
Psychotherapy to Peacemaking (1992)

Talking Back to Prozac: What Doctors Aren't
Telling You About Today's Most Controversial Drug (1994)
(Coauthored by Ginger Ross Breggin)

Psychosocial Approaches to Deeply Disturbed Persons (1996)
(Coedited by E. Mark Stern)

Brain-Disabling Treatments in Psychiatry: Drugs,
Electroshock and the Role of the FDA (1997)

The Heart of Being Helpful: Empathy
and the Creation of a Healing Presence (1997)

The War Against Children of Color: Psychiatry Targets
Inner-City Youth (1998) (Coauthored by Ginger Ross Breggin)

Your Drug May Be Your Problem: How and Why to Stop Taking
Psychiatric Medications (1999) (Coauthored by David Cohen)

Reclaiming Our Children: A Healing
Solution for a Nation in Crisis (2000)

Talking Back to Ritalin: What Doctors Aren't
Telling You About Stimulants for Children (rev. ed. 2001)

Fiction

The Crazy from the Sane (1971)
After the Good War (1972)

The
ANTIDEPRESSANT
FACT BOOK

What Your Doctor
Won't Tell You About
Prozac, Zoloft, Paxil, Celexa,
and Luvox

PETER R. BREGGIN, MD

Da Capo

LIFE
LONG

A Member of the Perseus Books Group

To my editor, Marnie Cochran,
and to my agent, Andrew Blauner

Copyright © 2001 by Peter R. Breggin

Cataloging-in-Publication Data is available from the Library of Congress.
ISBN 0-7382-0451-X

Da Capo Press is a member of the Perseus Books Group.

Da Capo Press books are available at special discounts for bulk purchases in the U.S. by corporations, institutions, and other organizations. For more information, please contact the Special markets Department at the Perseus Books Group, 11 Cambridge Center, Cambridge, MA 02142, or call (800) 255-1415 or email special.markets@perseusbooks.com.

Find us on the World Wide Web at http://www.dacapopress.com
Text design by Elizabeth Lahey
Set in 10.5-point Sabon by Perseus Publishing Services

First printing, July 2001

5 6 7 8 9 10 - 06 05 04

Contents

THREE

FOUR

Contents / vii

EIGHT

NINE

TEN

ELEVEN

TWELVE

SIXTEEN

A Reader Alert

The *Antidepressant Fact Book* is about depression—how to think about and treat it. The focus is on the newer antidepressants, especially the SSRIs, and how they affect the brain and mind. The goal is to bring you facts that you will not find in other sources.

The SSRIs, with their chemical names in parentheses, include:

> Prozac and Sarafem (fluoxetine)
> Zoloft (sertraline)
> Paxil (paroxetine)
> Celexa (citalopram)
> Luvox (fluvoxamine)

The book will also discuss other relatively new antidepressants, especially in comparison with the SSRIs, including Effexor (venlafaxine), Serzone (nefazodone), Wellbutrin or Zyban (buproprion), and Remeron (mirtazapine).

Antidepressants are not only dangerous to use, withdrawal reactions can make them dangerous to stop taking. Especially when used for more than a few weeks or in larger doses, they can cause potentially severe withdrawal reactions, including anxiety, depression, and suicidal feelings. It is best to withdraw from these drugs gradually and with the help of an experienced professional.

No book can substitute for a clinical evaluation or experienced professional help, but this book will provide you information that is unavailable anywhere else. It can make you a much better informed consumer and help you choose for yourself between the conflicting claims being made by professionals about how to deal with depression.

Acknowledgments

My assistant, Ian Goddard, has been very helpful in searching out new scientific material and in editing several of the chapters. My senior editor, Marnie Cochran, and my project editor, Marco Pavia, remain as wonderful as ever. I cannot thank my agent, Andrew Blauner, enough for his support.

My wife, Ginger, continues to inspire and help me in everything I do. With each succeeding publication, I try to find another way to express my gratitude to her for how she infuses all of my life with spirit and intelligence, as well as just plain help. I grow speechless with the effort of thanking her.

Finally, I want to thank Kevin McCready, Ph. D., for his helpful editing, but even more so for his contributions as the founder and director of the San Joaquin Psychotherapy Clinic in Clovis, California. Dr. McCready's clinic is unique in helping people withdraw from psychiatric drugs and in providing drug-free treatment for even the most difficult and distressed individuals. His dedication and courage in developing the San Joaquin Psychotherapy Clinic have established a higher standard for the entire profession.

Introduction:
Drug Facts You Cannot Get
Anywhere Else

Tens of millions of people have turned to a new class of antidepressants that now includes Prozac, Zoloft, Paxil, Celexa, and Luvox. These drugs are called SSRIs—Selective Serotonin Reuptake Inhibitors—because of their action on the neurotransmitter or chemical messenger named serotonin. Prozac, Zoloft and Paxil are among the largest selling drugs in the world.

In 2000 the manufacturer of Prozac, Eli Lilly and Co., claimed that more than 35 million people worldwide had taken their antidepressant drug. In the previous year, Prozac had generated more than one-quarter of the company's $10 billion in revenue. Prozac, Zoloft, and Paxil are among the top-selling drugs in the United States, with total sales exceeding $4 billion per year.[1]

The drug companies who manufacture and sell these drugs are so wealthy and powerful that they can influence and sometimes direct the basic institutions of our society. As a result, promotion for the SSRI "antidepressants" has changed the way many people view themselves when they become depressed. In response to an enormously expensive and successful marketing campaign, more and more people think that depression is biochemical and that they ought to try one or more of these drugs if they feel depressed.

Too Little Skepticism

Most Americans realize that the manufacturers and distributors of consumer goods cannot be trusted to inform the public about all the dangers involved in using their products. The public was recently treated to the sight of televised congressional hearings at which the Ford Motor Company and Firestone Tire Co. executives pointed their fingers at each other in regard to the deadly rollovers that have afflicted the Ford Explorer. Ford blamed faulty tires and Firestone blamed faulty automobiles. Sophisticated citizens probably didn't fully believe either one of them.

Most Americans also realize that corporations try to bamboozle them with advertising into trusting and wanting their products. When they see an advertisement with a baby securely surrounded by a Michelin tire, they are under no illusion that the tire maker is more interested in their child's safety than in their dollars.

Similarly, most Americans were not surprised when it turned out that the tobacco companies were withholding information about the dangers of smoking or that the asbestos companies were trying to silence fears about their cancer-causing insulation. No one is shocked that the government has to force public utilities to stop polluting or alcoholic beverage manufactures to put warnings on their cans. Overall, we're a rather sophisticated citizenry with a fairly high index of suspicion about the products we buy and the corporations that influence our lives.

But something happens to us when we are dealing with companies that make prescription medicines. Perhaps it's the aura of FDA approval. Perhaps it's the passage of these drugs through the trusted hands of our physicians. Perhaps it's the cleverness of the ad campaigns. Perhaps we just can't believe that anyone would sell poison as if it were a miracle cure. But in reality—much like automobiles, tobacco, and asbestos products—psychiatric drugs are products sold in a competitive marketplace. This book aims, above all else, to encourage a healthy skepticism toward the claims made for antidepressant drugs.

Unique Sources of Information

Many books have been written about these new "antidepressants," but this book provides detailed information that is unavailable elsewhere. The same drug companies that have the power to influence the values of our society also have the power to influence drug research and its outcome, as well as the views of most professionals who write about or prescribe the drugs.[2]

Facts, research, and science in the field of psychiatric drugs too often aren't what they seem to be, and the experts who write, lecture, and prescribe aren't always who they seem to be. Almost all the research is paid for by drug companies and nearly all the psychiatric drug experts are beholden to these corporations, often receiving money as consultants or researchers. These experts get paid to carry out studies on behalf of the companies, and they give seminars and write articles to promote their products. Most of them have relationships with several different drug companies. Often their university departments or research centers are dependent on drug-company funding.

In contrast to most experts in the field of psychiatric medications, I have an independent perspective, as well as sources of information unavailable to even the most sophisticated, experienced authorities in the field.

My work as a medical expert in court cases provides me sources of information about antidepressants that are unavailable to other experts in the field. The most dramatic findings have come from my work as a medical expert in cases brought against pharmaceutical companies by individuals who have been damaged by drugs.

Unlike the overwhelming majority of experts in the field, I have freed myself of drug company influence and the vested interests of organized psychiatry. Since leaving a full-time post at the National Institute of Mental Health (NIMH) in 1968, I have been in private practice as a psychiatrist. My private practice income has made me professionally and economically independent. Because I don't have any "employers" other than my clinical patients and my medical-legal clients, I don't have to withhold scientific truth to placate employers such as drug companies, psychiatric associations, research centers, medical schools, or clinics. I also don't take any money from drug companies, even when it's been offered to me for giving lectures to medical schools or hospitals.

As the director of the International Center for the Study of Psychiatry and Psychology for nearly three decades, I am the recipient of a constant flow of information from consumers and professionals around the world concerning the effects of psychiatric medications. As founder and coeditor of the center's peer-review journal, *Ethical Human Sciences and Services,* I keep in touch with the latest happenings in the field. In addition, I am routinely asked to give seminars to professional and lay audiences throughout North America and Europe concerning drugs. Finally, as the author of multiple books and peer-reviewed articles on psychiatric medication, I have reviewed and evaluated thousands of research books and articles over the past several decades.

Getting Inside the Drug Companies

I have learned the most about the real nature of antidepressants as a result of my ability as a medical expert to look inside the records of drug companies. I first became significantly involved in the medical-legal arena in the early 1970s as a medical expert in a trial that helped to stop the resurgence of lobotomy and other forms of psychosurgery. In the early 1990s my involvement in these forensic activities escalated after I was asked by a consortium of attorneys to become the medical expert in a large series of combined lawsuits against Eli Lilly and Co. concerning Prozac. I worked largely by myself for a year or more developing the scientific basis for hundreds of suits against the company that revolved around charges that Prozac causes violence, suicide, and psychosis. I continue to be consulted as an expert in various kinds of legal actions involving SSRIs, including Prozac, Zoloft, Paxil, Celexa, and Luvox. In 2000, for example, I led attorneys into SmithKline and Beecham's corporate headquarters outside Philadelphia to go through their files on Paxil and at the start of 2001 I was doing the same thing at Eli Lilly and Co. in Indianapolis regarding Prozac.

The legal process of obtaining otherwise secret information from the corporation is called "discovery." If a case against a corporation has merit, the judge can force the company to release all of its relevant records to the attorneys who have brought the suit. The lawyers then ask me to help them evaluate voluminous records with the aim of finding out if the company has been involved in negligent or fraudulent activities.

The documents are stacked in cartons that line walls and fill conference tables, sometimes in a room as large a small house. I look at secret corporate documents—everything from internal memos discussing how to suppress public and professional criticism to secret FDA warning letters about improper research procedures. There are dozens of cartons of materials that describe clinical trials and a wall of boxes that contain thousands of reports of adverse drug effects. There will be secret company reviews of the drug's efficacy and safety and discussions of marketing strategies.

The lawsuits in which I'm an expert vary widely in their nature. Many are product liability suits in which I am a medical expert for the plaintiff, typically an injured patient who was damaged by drugs. If the patient died, the family may bring the suit. Eli Lilly and Company, for example, has been sued hundreds of times for allegedly being negligent and fraudulent in the testing, development, and marketing of Prozac. Although I've been directly involved in only a fraction of these hundreds of legal actions, my research has probably provided the basis for most of them.

Eli Lilly and Co. has secretly and quietly settled many and probably most of these suits. With one exception among hundreds of cases, the company has not gone to court and won a suit. The exception was a case in Hawaii that was lost by the plaintiffs. I didn't participate in that case.

In another example of a suit involving SSRI antidepressants, I'm a medical expert in a product liability suit against SmithKline Beecham Pharmaceuticals concerning Paxil. A man drowned himself and his two children shortly after starting to take Paxil, and his family is suing the company for allegedly withholding information about Paxil's causing or exacerbating suicide and violence. I'm also a medical expert in a California business and professions fraud suit against the same company for allegedly failing to inform the public about severe withdrawal effects when trying to stop taking Paxil. In yet another suit, I am investigating the case of a young woman who burned herself to death after being prescribed Celexa.

All of these activities give me an inside track to factual information unavailable to other doctors.

Hiding the Facts

After so many revelations about corporations deceiving the public regarding the safety of their products, it should be no surprise that many pharmaceutical companies do the same thing. In reviewing the internal documents of Eli Lilly and Co., I found enormously important information that the corporation purposely withheld from the FDA and from the medical profession. I also found innumerable deviations from sound and ethical scientific practices. I have written about many aspects of this negligence in *Talking Back to Prozac* (with Ginger Breggin, 1994) and then updated the data in *Brain-Disabling Treatments in Psychiatry* (1997). This book will provide new disclosures as well.

I discovered, for example, that Prozac's manufacturer had systematically mislabeled many kinds of adverse reactions that patients were undergoing so that they would be hidden from view. A suicide by a patient taking Prozac could be filed away under the heading "no drug effect" or "depression." When the FDA or anyone else then examined the rates of suicide on patients taking Prozac, those patient suicides would never be counted, because a computer search would identify them as "no drug effect" or "depression" rather than "suicide."

I documented how the company manipulated its own clinical trials so that Prozac would come out looking better and less harmful than it was. I found secret studies the company had conducted that showed increased rates of overstimulation and suicide attempts on Prozac during controlled clinical trials (discussed in Chapters 2 and 3).

I also examined FDA reports and correspondence about Prozac that the government agency refused to disclose in response to freedom of information requests. Later on, I will describe how the FDA found that it was receiving unusually and disproportionately high rates of reported violence on Prozac (Chapter 4).

Quietly Settling the Cases

On a few occasions, I've testified in court against drug companies, including once against Eli Lilly and Co., but in the vast majority of cases, the companies settle out of court with as little publicity as possible. In fact, Eli Lilly and Co. has settled dozens and perhaps hundreds of lawsuits about Prozac without going to court. In every one of my cases, Eli Lilly and Co. has settled, including the only occasion when I testified in court against the corporation. As it was later proven and then admitted, Eli Lilly and Co. rigged the outcome of the jury trial by paying untold millions of dollars to the plaintiffs before the trial ended. In return, the plaintiffs pulled their legal punches. In other words, the drug company paid off the plaintiffs to cooperate in creating a fake courtroom drama that guaranteed a favorable outcome for the drug company.

It may seem unbelievable and even preposterous that Eli Lilly and Co. has sufficient power and influence to manipulate a trial to come out to its own advantage. It may also seem unbelievable these events have never been reported in major media. I will therefore describe the circumstances in some detail in Chapter 15 on SSRI-induced violence. For now, I want to challenge the commonplace assumption that the public and the health professions have access to reliable information about psychiatric drugs such as Prozac, Zoloft, Paxil, Celexa, and Luvox. To the contrary, they are exposed to an unrelenting, carefully orchestrated marketing campaign.

In my experience, psychiatrists and other physicians have very little knowledge about the limited testing involved in the FDA approval of drugs. Nor do they know much about how antidepressants impact their patients' brains or minds. In debates with my colleagues, I've heard statements like the following:

"FDA approval means that a drug is safe."
"The FDA makes sure that a drug is tested on thousands of patients before it is approved."
"Antidepressants are not mood-altering, they directly improve the disease of depression."
"Antidepressants are like insulin for diabetes, they provide essential missing substances."
"Antidepressants don't cause abnormalities in the brain, they correct biochemical imbalances."
"Antidepressants aren't in any way similar to stimulants like amphetamine and cocaine."
"Antidepressants don't cause withdrawal problems; you can stop them without any ill effects."
"Antidepressants can't make you psychotic unless you have a preexisting mental illness."

None of the above is true.

These, and many other myths and misunderstandings about depression and antidepressants, will be addressed in this book.

ONE

The Meaning and Purpose of Depression

For many centuries people have sought to overcome depression through both medical and psychological or spiritual means. The use of herbs, for example, St. John's wort, goes back at least to the Middle Ages. The use of religion and other spiritual approaches to depression goes back to the origins of humanity. Before written history, human beings conducted ritual burials of their dead that helped them deal with the painful feelings caused by bereavement. Depression is obviously part of the fabric of human experience—but what is it?

Depression is a psychological state—an emotional response to life. In particular, it is a feeling of hopelessness and despair that's often accompanied by self-hate and self-blame. These feelings can vary from barely perceptible to overwhelming. They can last for moments or for a lifetime.

Most people have experienced some degree of depressed feelings at one time or another, usually during and after great frustrations, disappointments, or losses. Many have felt "blue" or "sad" for significant portions of their lives. Usually these feelings go away with time, improved circumstances, and new approaches to making a successful life.

Unfortunately, some people end up feeling trapped in an unendurable depressed state of mind. Feeling that they do not deserve to live or that they have no viable options for happiness, they become emotionally paralyzed and suicidal. In desperation, they will accept almost any kind of treatment that offers hope of relief. Other people seem to live for many years or most of their lives with lingering feelings of sadness that never seem to go away.

Mild feelings of depression are a part of routine living, but even more painful feelings of depression are common. Surveys indicate that one in five people at some time will experience a depressed state of mind that noticeably impairs their ability to enjoy life or to take care of themselves. Although there is good reason to distrust these surveys—they are usually conducted for the purpose of promoting biological psychiatry and drugs—they nonetheless reflect the reality that many people feel depressed at one time or another. Indeed, feelings of depression are even more common among adolescents, the elderly, women, and other vulnerable groups. Feeling depressed plays a significant part in the lives of many if not most people at some point in their lifetime.

The Most Common Causes of Depressed Feelings

Most people who seek help for depression have experienced distressing recent events such as a failing or conflicted marriage, a series of broken love relationships, or a disrupted career. Sometimes they are grieving the death of a loved one. Others feel depressed over their struggle with chronic physical pain or alcoholism and drug addiction. Some have become depressed after being told they have a serious illness or while recuperating from open-heart surgery. Other people seek help for lifelong feelings of depression that can be traced back to childhood neglect and abuse or to losses and disappointments in early adulthood.

When most people seek help from a psychiatrist or other mental health professionals, the sources of their depressed feelings are readily apparent. Rarely do people seek help for a depression that has come upon them "out of the blue" or for no apparent reason at all. They may start out the first consultation by saying or even believing that there's no apparent cause for their suffering, but a few thoughtful inquiries usually reveal that they know what's upsetting them but cannot bear to think and talk about it.

Mired Down in Depressed Feelings

Depression is such a dreadful experience that most people will do almost anything to get rid of the painful feelings. Many lapse into an emotional dullness in an attempt to escape their suffering. Some end up committing suicide. Others allow doctors to blunt their minds and damage their brains with drugs or electroshock.

Although they desperately want to get better, persistently depressed people tend to be stuck with self-defeating ideas about life. They are prevented from seeking self-fulfillment or happiness by their conflicts and their misguided approaches to living. Almost always, they have given up making their dreams come true. They "sacrifice" for others without really making anyone happy. Worst of all, they no longer feel they can make meaningful or satisfying choices. They cannot see a positive way to influence the course of their lives. They feel utterly helpless. Indeed, they are overwhelmed by feelings of helplessness.

A man who has been raised to believe that divorce is morally and religiously prohibited may become depressed if he feels he cannot have a satisfactory life without divorcing. If he has been taught to feel guilty about even desiring a better marriage, he will be especially vulnerable to depression.

I am not suggesting that people who hold marriage to be inviolable are more depression prone. Viewing marriage as inviolable could also provide the basis for a very satisfying life. However, paralyzing conflict between religious values learned in childhood and personal desires in adulthood commonly leads to feelings of depression.

Similarly, a woman who believes her "place is in the home" may derive great satisfaction from being a wife and homemaker. But she is likely to become vulnerable to depression when she develops conflicting values about her own self-fulfillment through alternative directions, such as going to college or becoming a professional.

The Special Vulnerability of Depressed Children

In my practice I treat individual adults, couples, and children with their families. Working with children and their families provides an open window into how and why people become depressed. A child can become depressed by the death of a parent, the divorce of parents, sexual or emotional abuse, school failure, or peer abuse in school. Often children are depressed by simply not receiving all the love and attention they need from busy and stressed parents. At yet other times, they become depressed over the unrelenting boredom and alienation they feel at school. At other times, they become depressed because the family, the school, the church, and the community have failed to give them the kind of moral and spiritual direction that children need to lead meaningful lives.

Parents have been losing their influence over their children. The school experience has loomed larger and larger. So has the peer group. Indeed, some of the more profound suffering among children results from abuse by other children who ridicule and ostracize them.

Despite the increasing disempowerment of parents, mothers and fathers remain the single most important source of healing in the lives of children. If the parents work together to provide understanding, consistent love, and rational discipline to an emotionally injured child, recovery can often take place almost overnight, and improvement can always begin immediately.

Nowadays psychiatric drugs, including stimulants like Ritalin and Adderall, commonly cause children to become depressed.[1] When doctors fail to recognize the drug-induced nature of the child's depression, they mistakenly prescribe antidepressants that worsen the child's mental condition. This leads to further deterioration, more drugs, and increased blunting of the child's mental life. By the time I become involved as a "psychiatrist of last resort," drugs have taken the luster out of the child's eyes, and the child roller-coasters from one unstable emotion to another.

When Nothing Helps . . .

I often work with very depressed children and adults who have failed to "get better" despite years of treatment by other doctors. In these instances, I usually find one or more of the following circumstances:

- Years of treatment by authoritarian, uncaring doctors or therapists
- Years of exposure to multiple psychiatric drugs
- Long-term submission to an emotionally abusive parent, spouse, or loved one

Especially in recent years, the individual's previous doctors may have overlooked or denied the obvious harmful effects of severe emotional, physical or sexual abuse in childhood.

My task as a psychiatrist and psychotherapist is to help these desperate children and adults to recover from a series of oppressive relationships and from the harmful effects of their previous therapy and psychiatric drugs. My goal is to encourage better principles for taking care of themselves and their loved ones and to inspire them to pursue the kind of life that will bring them greater personal satisfaction and happiness.

Depressed people often feel very guilty about pursuing their own needs or desires, and although they may sacrifice for others, they usually resent it. However, during their recovery they rarely have to choose between selfishness and happiness. The pursuit of their ideals almost always brings out even greater potential to care for and to love other people, and to contribute to society in a more creative manner. I will discuss basic principles for better living in the final chapter of this book.

Not a Disease

It is a mistake to view depressed feelings or even severely depressed feelings as a "disease." Depression, remember, is an emotional response to life. It is a feeling of unhappiness—a particular kind of unhappiness that involves helpless self-blame and guilt, a sense of not deserving happiness, and a loss of interest in life. As already described, abused children almost always suffer unhappiness in the form of depressed feelings. So do adults who go through serious losses in regard to loved ones or employment. Chronic pain and ill health usually produce some degree of depressed feelings. In that sense, depression is a natural or normal human response to emotional injury and loss.

Even when depressed feelings become extreme or unrelenting, these reactions usually have obvious causes, such as the breakup of a marriage, the inability to leave an unhappy marriage, the death of a loved one, failure at work, an inability to achieve one's fondest hopes in life, ill health, or a lonely old age. A human emotional or psychological state—basically, a feeling—should not be considered a "disease" simply because it becomes extreme.

The term "antidepressant" should always be thought of with quotation marks around it because there is little or no reason to believe that these drugs target depression or depressed feelings. In fact, I find considerable evidence that these drugs have little or no therapeutic effect on feelings of depression.

So-called antidepressants in actual practice are being prescribed for many problems other than depression, including anxiety, panic, eating problems, premenstrual tension, stress, posttraumatic stress disorder, and obsessions and compulsions. They are being given to increasing numbers of children, including toddlers, despite studies showing how harmful and ineffective they are when given to children.

Is it possible that all of these various emotional and psychological problems are chemically related to one another and therefore responsive to one class of drugs that affects a specific brain chemical? Whatever effect these drugs have, we will have to look for a mechanism other than the correction of a "biochemical imbalance."

Even Whole Cultures

The psychological nature of depression is confirmed by the fact that whole groups of people and even societies can become largely depressed. Sometimes most of the people in a culture will become depressed. I was shocked to read an early account of Native American life in a southeastern nation. The Native Americans were described as emotionally expressive people who laughed and played a great deal. That's quite a different picture than we now have of Native Americans. Many Native American peoples developed their stoic demeanor in response to years of oppression that, in many cases, led to the extinction of entire nations.

I will never forget a brief visit I made to East Berlin before the Berlin Wall came down. Everywhere around me, the surroundings were depressing and the people, as a whole, seemed depressed. Awareness of what we are missing or prevented from having makes us especially vulnerable to depression, and the East Berliners knew about the greater opportunities that lay beyond their reach a few feet across the Berlin Wall. In addition, East Berliners under communism were taught that it was wrong to desire the "materialism" of the Western, capitalistic world, adding to their internal conflict and helpless feelings of depression.

Depression can also affect victimized groups within a culture. Many surveys have concluded that women are more prone to depression than men. This vulnerability results from the frequency and depth of the paralyzing conflicts that many women experience concerning their contradictory expectations and roles in modern society. Women also frequently end up taking on themselves the responsibilities for home and family that men too easily evade or forsake. Despite the advances that have been made in providing equal opportunity to women, they continue to run smack into unfair and unacknowledged limits on their choices in the home, workplace, and society. However, if women can identify the problem and overcome culturally built-in feelings of guilt, they can take as effective action as possible without lapsing into depression.

Depression is more common everywhere that choices and opportunities are stifled, and where people are taught that they do not deserve or cannot achieve anything better. In the United States depression is especially common among the poor, among oppressed minorities, in economically depressed communities, and among women, especially elderly women.

Depression Occurs in a Context

Unfortunately, the medical approach to depression has influenced many people to completely ignore the real bases for feeling depressed, including obvious societal and cultural cases. An article titled "Up from Depression" appeared in the February 2001 edition of the newspaper published by AARP, the American Association of Retired People. Surely this group should be sensitive to the real needs of the elderly, and indeed the report gives passing mention to the problems of infirmity, loneliness, and isolation among the old in America. But in response to a variety of medically oriented "experts," AARP ultimately comes out firmly for the biological view of depression. We are treated to quotes that affirm that depression is a "medical disorder, like hypertension or diabetes" and that "depression is an illness." Instead of increased professsional and volunteer services, instead of greater family and community involvement, instead of more overall appreciation of our older citizens, the article emphasizes the supposed value of antidepressant drugs and even electroshock.

Depression is not a "disorder" that can be separated from the context in which people live and make choices. Feeling depressed is a human response to circumstances that feel intolerable and from which the individual sees no possible escape. If the person also feels guilty and ashamed about personal desires for a better life, then depressed feelings are almost inevitable.

Selling "Depression" as a Disease

If you want to make people buy a product, you have to convince them that they want or need it. To market psychiatric drugs, people have to be convinced that they have "diseases" that can be "treated" with the drugs. As I'll document in later chapters, the word "depression" has come to mean a "disorder" or a "disease" by dint of aggressive marketing. In reality, depression is always recognized or identified on the basis of how an individual feels.

The 1856 *American Dictionary of the English Language* by Noah Webster defines *depression* as "a sinking of the spirits; dejection; a state of sadness; want of courage or animation; as depression of the mind." Webster defines *melancholy* as a severe form of depression. Melancholy is "a gloomy state of mind, often a gloomy state that is of some continuance, or habitual; depression of the spirits induced by grief; dejection of the spirits. This was formerly supposed to proceed from a redundance of black bile."

Webster's definition, nearly 150 years old, is remarkable for its use of ordinary moral, psychological, and even spiritual language to describe the facets of feeling depressed, and for its recognition of the relationship between depressed feelings and grief. Webster's observation that melancholy was "formerly supposed to proceed from a redundance of black bile" reminds us that medicine and psychiatry have for hundreds of years offered mistaken ideas about the biological origin of feelings of depression. In the future,

I am hopeful, definitions will declare that depression was "formerly supposed to proceed from a biochemical imbalance." Unfortunately, however, the biochemical myth—unlike the bile myth—has the power of a billion-dollar industry behind it.

The definition of depression has changed little over the centuries. The 2000 *Stedman's Medical Dictionary* defines depression as "characterized by feelings of sadness, loneliness, despair, low self-esteem and self-reproach." The 2000 *Dorland's Illustrated Medical Dictionary* says that depression is "characterized by feelings of sadness, despair, and discouragement." It compares depression to the "the blues" and to "bereavement," and adds, "there are often feelings of low self-esteem, guilt, and self-reproach." Thus, even the medical dictionaries confirm that depression is an emotional state that is familiar to everyone and readily described in everyday language.

Depression is never defined by an objective physical finding, such as a blood test or brain scan. It is defined by the individual's personal suffering and especially by the depressed thoughts and feelings that the person expresses. In other words, if a person has depressed thoughts and feelings, the diagnosis of depression is made. Based on that alone, it makes little sense to view depressed feelings, or the emotional state of depression, as a disease or disorder.

The severity of a person's depression should not mislead one into thinking it is a genuine physical disease like diabetes or pneumonia. Depression is always defined by its subjective emotional quality. It can only be identified in terms of the person's feelings or through behaviors, such as a sad face or suicidal acts, that provide a window into that person's feelings.

The "Official" Definition of
Depression and *Antidepressant*

Even the 1856 Webster's dictionary was not free of medical influence. Its definition observed, "Melancholy, when extreme and of long continuance, is a disease sometimes accompanied with partial insanity." There was in 1856 no scientific basis for determining that sadness becomes a "disease" by dint of being extreme or persistent. There is still no reason to define grief, dejection, or melancholia as a "disease" simply because it is severe or lasting.

Although depression is experienced as emotional or psychological suffering, medically oriented scientists and practitioners have tried to redefine these feelings into something that looks more like a biological disorder. Toward this end, the official diagnostic manual of the American Psychiatric Association, the *Diagnostic and Statistical Manual of Mental Disorders IV* (1994), has attempted to formulate diagnostic categories for various experiences of depression. The categories are then used to frame depression as a medical disorder for purposes of promoting psychiatric drugs.

Antidepressants are psychoactive drugs that have been approved by the FDA for use in treating clinical depression or major depression, as defined by the official diagnostic manual. According to these criteria, clinical or major depression must include at least two weeks of "depressed mood" or "loss of interest of pleasure," as well as four other symptoms from a list that includes significant weight loss, insomnia, fatigue, agitation, feelings of worthlessness, and recurrent thoughts of death. The manual acknowledges that the person's mood is often described by the individual as "depressed, sad, hopeless, discouraged, or 'down in the dumps'." It also observes that depressed people often suffer from a sense of "worthlessness or guilt."

In other words, to fit the official diagnosis you have to be *unhappy in a depressed fashion* for two weeks. Why two weeks instead of one week, six weeks, or two months? There is no rational basis for determining how long a person is "allowed" to feel depressed before deserving a diagnosis. The authors of the definition needed a minimal time period to look more scientific so they made one up.

Unanswered Questions

Although it provides the basis for justifying the prescription of antidepressant drugs, the official diagnosis of major depression leaves many questions unanswered. Most important, it does not deal with why people get depressed. Is the person who feels sad after the death of a loved one suffering from the same "disorder" as the person who feels sad as a result of the emotionally depressing effects of a hormonal disorder or a medication? Is the person whose life is spiritually empty in the same diagnostic category as a person who is recovering from rape? Is the person who is depressed over irrational guilt from childhood in the same category as the person who is depressed after being caught and imprisoned for a remorseless crime? Is the child depressed by poverty, racism, or sexism the same as the child who is depressed by failing to maintain perfect grades the way his or her parents demand?

Is the man who is depressed over a lifelong relationship with an abusive parent the same as a man who is depressed over his failure to beat his wife into submission? Is the woman who is depressed over sexist oppression in her workplace the same as the woman who feels jealous and depressed over the success of other women?

Depression is a human response to a wide variety of psychological, spiritual, and even physical factors. It displays itself in myriad ways from chronic feelings of sadness to acute feelings of wanting to die. It drives some people to feel suicidal and others to feel murderous. It provides some people an excuse to be needy and demanding in relationships with other people, whereas it compels others to try to live even more independent lives.

It is misleading to lump everyone into the simplistic category of major depression. It becomes even more potentially harmful to assume that most or even all of these people should be treated with antidepressant drugs. Nonetheless, in actual practice, anyone with significantly depressed feelings is diagnosed with major depression and is almost certain to be treated with drugs and even electroshock.

From Bile to Biochemical Imbalances

As already noted, the biochemical imbalance theory is the natural heir of the bad bile theory of depression. Increasingly, there is a tendency among biological psychiatrists to view even mild, transient expressions of depression as biochemical in origin. Once again, this is the product of aggressive marketing and public relations efforts by organized psychiatry and pharmaceutical companies. The result is that 20 million or more Americans have tried antidepressants.

Medications aimed specifically at depression were first developed in the 1950s and resulted in renewed claims that depression is biological and caused by biochemical imbalances. Although it was relatively easy to disprove the bile mythology, the very vagueness of the biochemical imbalance theory has made it easy to imagine these imbalances without having to prove that they exist. Biological psychiatry advocates often do not even bother to name the particular biochemical that is supposedly out of balance, or they change the allegedly offending biochemical depending on what kind of drug they are pushing. In reality, science does not have the ability to measure the levels of any biochemical in the tiny spaces between nerve cells (the synapses) in the brain of a human being. All the talk about biochemical imbalances is sheer speculation aimed at promoting psychiatric drugs.

The Search for Biological Markers for Depression

Biological advocates claim that depression is a physical disease because it can cause physical symptoms. Physicians, including psychiatrists like myself, are trained to focus on the body rather than the mind or the spirit. As a result, many of us tend to confuse the physical results of depression with the primary problem of feeling depressed.

Weight loss, which is called a "vegetative sign" of depression, is a good example of this confusion. People who are depressed often lose their interest in feeling pleasure, including their appetite for food. They may even lose their desire to keep themselves alive by eating. Naturally, they lose weight. Biological psychiatrists often cite weight loss as a so-called vegetative or physical sign of depression, but weight loss is not specific to depression at all. In fact, some people tend to eat more when they are depressed. When weight loss does occur during depression, it's usually the result of not caring to eat.

Similarly, psychomotor retardation is used as a physical sign of depression. Psychomotor retardation refers to the fact that depressed, discouraged people will often begin to think, speak, and to walk more slowly. We've all seen friends or family act that way when "feeling down." You can see it every weekend on television at the end of football, baseball, or basketball games. The winners jump around and talk so fast that they get breathless. It's their expression of joy. The losers, in dramatic contrast, walk off slowly with their heads bowed and with seemingly little interest in talking. It's an expression of sadness in response to losing. Doctors refer to these physical expressions of sadness as psychomotor retardation, but that doesn't make them symptoms of a medical disorder. They are expressions of feeling so sad and unhappy that nothing else seems to matter anymore.

Attempts have also been made to find physical markers for depression, the equivalent of lab tests that indicate liver disease or a recent heart attack. Despite decades of research, thousands of research studies, and hundreds of millions of dollars in expense, no marker for depression has been found. To this day, the individual's personal feelings remain the basis for diagnosing depression. When we speak of depression we mean a feeling about oneself and life.

Of course, the intensity of depressed feelings, like any emotion, can vary from very mild to very strong but the subjective experience remains basically the same. Human suffering can become extreme without being biological or genetic in origin. The most painful feelings in human life are the result of life experiences, such as the death of loved ones and the collapse of a marriage.

The PET Scan Scam

Biological psychiatry advocates like to show brain scans of depressed people as if they are somehow different from those of other people. In fact, doctors cannot diagnose depression from a brain scan because there are no consistent differences from "normal" brain scans. If depressed brain scans showed differences, such as a reduced metabolic rate in the frontal lobes, it would by no means demonstrate a biological cause. Far more likely, it would indicate that depressed feelings produce a flattening of emotional activity and hence brain activity. It is similar to the condition of a muscle that isn't being exercised; its metabolism will be much lower than that of a muscle that is being exercised.

An enormous multicolor ad for Prozac takes up the entire eighteen-by-twelve-inch back page of the January 19, 2001, edition of *Psychiatric News,* the official newspaper of the American Psychiatric Association. Most of the ad is taken up by the side view of the head of a smiling woman whose brain is portrayed as a fiery red, green, and yellow rendition of a brain scan. The page blazes with the message that depressed people have an abnormal brain scan that is made normal, or even better than normal, by Prozac.

Buried in the woman's hair in tiny print is the following statement: "This image is an adaptation of a PET scan of a normal brain. Prior history of depression is unknown." This in effect confesses, "We're intentionally giving you the wrong impression. Brain scans have nothing to do with depression and Prozac." FDA regulations on truth and fairness in advertising undoubtedly required this disclaimer but the advertisement's impact is hardly truthful or fair.

If the Drugs "Work," It's Biological

Nowadays it's common to claim that the effectiveness of drugs proves the biological origin of depression. Chapter 12 will find ample reason to question the efficacy of antidepressants. However, the seeming effectiveness of a psychoactive drug by no means indicates that it is addressing an underlying medical problem. Human beings have used alcohol, coca leaves (cocaine), and a variety of herbs for thousands of years to alleviate emotional suffering, including feelings of depression or melancholy. The fact that a drug such as alcohol or cocaine can relieve sadness or other painful emotions such as anxiety or chronic anger in no way indicates that the painful emotional state has a biological origin.

Many men drink alcohol to overcome their disappointment when their favorite team loses a game. They also drink alcohol to overcome the larger frustrations and stresses of life. Many women take uppers and downers to get through the stress and disappointment of their family lives. An enormous variety of prescription and over-the-counter drugs, as well as illegal drugs, seem to help many people to relieve a wide range of emotional suffering. But the relief tends to be temporary, and the drug often ends up causing more harm than good. Meanwhile, the psychoactive effects of these or any other drugs—including their tendency to cause emotional anesthesia or artificial euphoria—do not depend on an underlying biological cause.

The Meaning and Purpose of Depression

Most people come to medical and mental health professionals for help with depressed feelings that have readily discernible causes in the frustrations, conflicts, and losses they have endured. Only on occasion do we have to dig very deeply to discover why someone has become despairing over his or her life. However, even when the sources of the depressed feelings are obvious, overcoming them can be difficult. When life has driven a person to feel overwhelmingly helpless and despairing, it may take time and effort to find the understanding, direction, motivation, and courage to climb out of the depressed outlook.

It can become nearly impossible to rise out of depression on one's own—to "pull yourself up by your bootstraps." At times of great despair, people need people. A caring therapist, a loved one, or a devoted community such as an extended family or church can be lifesaving. But when a doctor spends fifteen minutes with his patient and prescribes a drug, the sense of aloneness and isolation is likely to be reinforced. The very idea of turning to pills instead of people can add to the feelings of despair and hopelessness. In short, it is depressing to believe that an improved life is best achieved by taking a pill.

Despite the claims of modern psychiatry, there is no checklist with which to determine that you have a disorder that can be treated with drugs. There is no magic bullet medication that can target your depression and cure it for you. Ultimately, each of us has a unique life story, and our own reasons for why we feel the way we do. There is no substitute for confronting how and why our lives have become so depressing to us. There is no satisfactory alternative to changing our approach to life as a way of overcoming or transcending depression.

Most people who seek help for depression have no idea that their feelings of depression actually have a purpose in their lives. But when the meaning and purpose of depression are understood, the individual can actually benefit from the experience.

Depression is, above all else, a signal that our lives are not going well. Emotional pain should direct our attention to the source of the suffering and motivate us to face the conflicts and stresses in our lives, including the ones that have seemed too painful to think about. Remember that the depth of our despair often reflects the contrasting desire that we have to live a more joyful, creative, and meaningful life. I often explain to my patients that they should be encouraged by the intensity of their psychological suffering because it confirms the depth of their feeling about life and their potential to bring enormous energy to a more constructive approach to living. If they did not strongly desire a much more fulfilling life, they wouldn't be so despairing over the one that they have. I then try to help them to locate the sources of the suffering and to work toward the creation of a genuinely satisfying and even wonderful life. In this way, feeling depressed can become an important stage in confronting an unhappy life and in building a better one.

Impairing our emotional awareness and our intellectual acuity with psychoactive drugs such as the SSRI antidepressants tends to impede the process of overcoming depression. We need all the resources of a fully functioning brain in order to plumb the depths of our emotions, to find the sources of both the suffering and the potential for joy, and to build a life based on principled living and happiness.

TWO

Damaging the Brain with SSRI Antidepressants

Our society looks upon psychiatric drugs with such naive trust that when an illegal drug can be compared to a psychiatric drug, it raises the illegal drug's social and medical status. Thus, a personal account in the January 21, 2001, *New York Times Magazine* praises the street stimulant "Ecstasy"[1] as a "whopper of an antidepressant" that's better than Prozac.[2] The author then blames the government for funding research that documents the brain-damaging effect of Ecstasy. After all, he reminds us, "Prozac-style antidepressants produce some morphological [structural] abnormalities in the serotonin nerve network of rats that resemble changes seen with Ecstasy taken in high levels. Yet few people advocate the banning of Prozac."

The Ecstasy advocate is right that government health agencies are eager to show that illegal drugs cause brain damage at the same time they resist informing the public that SSRI antidepressants do the same thing. He's also right that the same kind of research that is used to justify a ban on Ecstasy could potentially be used to justify a ban on SSRI antidepressants. However, he comes to the wrong conclusion. His observations should make him concerned about the dangers of both Ecstasy and the Prozac-like drugs. Consistent with society's infatuation with psychiatric substances, he instead makes more outlandish claims for Ecstasy.

The worship of Ecstasy is reminiscent of Freud's ecstatic enthusiasm for cocaine that ended in addiction and mental impairment for him and for those who believed him.[3] Closer to home, it's also reminiscent of the LSD craze of the 1960s that left many people with permanent harmful effects.

The Myth That Millions of Users Are Living Proof of a Drug's Safety

People understandably tend to think that a medication must be safe if it's been used by large numbers of people for many years. However, alcohol and tobacco were used as psychoactive drugs by hundreds of millions of people for hundreds and even thousands of years before their adverse effects became more apparent in recent decades. Similarly, psychiatric drugs can be used for a long time without their dangers being recognized.

As I will describe in chapter 4, neuroleptic or antipsychotic drugs produce an extremely high rate of relatively obvious and sometimes disabling abnormal movements, including spasms and contortions. Studies have shown, for example, that more than 50 percent of state hospital patients had symptoms of drug-induced tardive dyskinesia.[4] Yet the movement disorder remained almost unrecognized in the medical and psychiatric profession for the first twenty years of neuroleptic use from 1954 through 1973. Today many doctors continue to underestimate the risk.

Drugs can be on the market for decades or longer before their adverse effects cause the FDA to demand their withdrawal from the market. In 1997 the diet drugs fenfluramine (Pondimin) and dexfenfluramine (Redux) were withdrawn from the market by the FDA because they cause cardiac valve abnormalities.[5] Pondimin had been approved by the FDA approximately twenty-five years earlier. It had been given to millions of patients in the

intervening time for weight management. In addition to the cardiac valve problems, fenfluramines were also known to produce
a potentially fatal disorder called primary pulmonary hypertension and could have been withdrawn from the market on that
basis alone. Furthermore, for several decades evidence had been
accumulating that the fenfluramines, including dexfenfluramine,
destroy brain cells and chronically impair mental function.[6] They
are among the most neurotoxic drugs ever approved for use in
the United States, but the medical and psychiatric profession
showed shockingly little concern about permanently damaging
the brains of their patients.

The use of a psychiatric drug by millions of people for many
years by no means guarantees either the effectiveness or the safety
of the drug. This chapter will examine SSRI-induced brain damage and dysfunction in greater detail than is elsewhere available.
Because the FDA does not require adequate studies of the brain-
damaging effects of psychiatric drugs before their approval, and
because drug companies discourage such research, much of the
data presented in this chapter will be drawn from a variety of
studies conducted outside the drug companies within recent years.

Closely Related Drugs

Prozac is the trade name for fluoxetine, a chemical invented in a
laboratory by the pharmaceutical firm Eli Lilly and Co. The FDA
approved Prozac for marketing in the United States in December
1987. Other drug companies followed suit with SSRIs such as
Zoloft, Paxil, Celexa, and Luvox. Luvox is approved in the
United States for treating obsessive-compulsive disorder, but not
depression. None of these drugs are approved for the treatment
of depression in children.

Prozac, Zoloft, Paxil, Celexa, and Luvox are so similar that
for most purposes they can be discussed together. When occasionally necessary, distinctions will be made among them. Many
other of the newer antidepressants such as Effexor and Serzone

also share many characteristics with the SSRIs, especially their dangerous stimulating effects and the paradoxical tendency to cause depression.

Recently, a "new" form of Prozac was under development but had to be canceled at the last minute owing to adverse effects on the heart. I will look at the implications of this when I consider cardiovascular problems caused by SSRIs.

How SSRIs Work

The new antidepressants are called SSRIs. SSRI stands for Selective Serotonin Reuptake Inhibitor. The concept is not as complicated as it sounds. Serotonin is a neurotransmitter or chemical messenger that is released by one nerve cell or neuron to make another neuron fire. The serotonin is released into the synapse, or space between the neurons. In the natural course of events, the serotonin is then chemically destroyed or reabsorbed back into the cell that originally released it. But SSRI antidepressants block the reabsorption (reuptake) of the serotonin, causing an excess amount of serotonin to accumulate in the synapse. With more serotonin in the synapse, the theory suggests, the activity of the system will increase.

The Nature of Serotonin

Serotonin is a chemical distributed throughout the human body. When it was also found to function as a neurotransmitter in the brain, Eli Lilly and Co. decided to make a drug aimed at increasing the activity of serotonin in the brain.

The drug company was inspired by highly theoretical speculations about the role of serotonin in the brain. Many but not all drugs used to treat feelings of depression seem to artificially jack up the activity of chemical messengers such as acetylcholine, norepinephrine, and dopamine, as well as serotonin. Eli Lilly and Co. anticipated that creating a drug to selectively stimulate serotonin nerve transmission would result in a marketable antidepressant. Company researchers synthesized and tested a variety of chemicals before finding one that would selectively interfere with the removal of serotonin from the synapse.

Limits of the Serotonin Theory

The theory is simple enough, but the reality of brain function is much more complex and shrouded in mystery. Synapses are tiny spaces between neurons that are too small to be seen with an ordinary microscope. There are trillions of synapses in the brain, many filled with a souplike mixture of innumerable chemicals.

Each nerve cell manufactures, stores, and periodically releases one or more chemical messengers into the synapse. These chemicals attach to nearby cells to make them fire. Neurotransmitters are like sparks that ignite the flash pans of other neurons. When sufficient numbers of these chemical messengers attach to a cell, the cell fires (see Figure 2.1). All neurons have receptors on their surfaces that are tailored to receive specific chemical messengers. In regard to serotonin, there are many different types and subtypes of receptors, and more continue to be discovered. Their functions in the brain are not understood.

Serotonin is one of hundreds of chemicals that affect brain function. Almost nothing is known about the relationships among the hundreds of millions of neurons and these chemicals, and equally little is known about their relationship to the overall function of the mind or the brain.

The Complexity of the Serotonin System

Tampering with the serotonin neurotransmitter system is especially fraught with difficulties because the serotonin nerves spread in a vast network through the brain (Figure 2.2). Essentially, they go everywhere.

The serotonin nerve bodies are clustered together in the lower part of the brain called the raphe nuclei. Their extensions, called axons, spread out throughout the entire brain. They end up stimulating other neurons in every lobe of the brain, as well as cells in the pituitary gland. Of all the neurotransmitter systems that

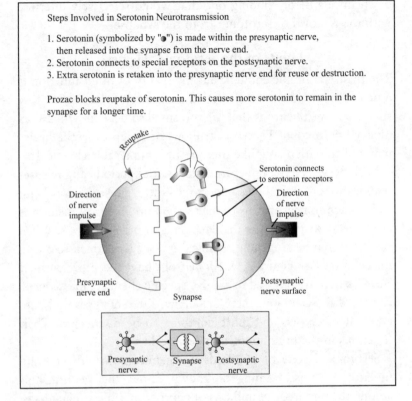

Steps Involved in Serotonin Neurotransmission

1. Serotonin (symbolized by "●") is made within the presynaptic nerve, then released into the synapse from the nerve end.
2. Serotonin connects to special receptors on the postsynaptic nerve.
3. Extra serotonin is retaken into the presynaptic nerve end for reuse or destruction.

Prozac blocks reuptake of serotonin. This causes more serotonin to remain in the synapse for a longer time.

Reuptake

Serotonin connects to serotonin receptors

Direction of nerve impulse

Direction of nerve impulse

Presynaptic nerve end

Postsynaptic nerve surface

Synapse

Presynaptic nerve

Synapse

Postsynaptic nerve

FIGURE 2.1

have been studied, the network of serotonin neurons is the most widespread.

Overall, the functioning of the serotonin system is complex beyond our imagination. Science has hardly stuck its big toe into this ocean, and yet biopsychiatry avidly continues to recruit millions of patients into what is essentially an out-of-control societal experiement.

Disrupting the Serotonin System

Despite our inability to understand the complexity or functions of this or any other neurotransmitter, we do know something

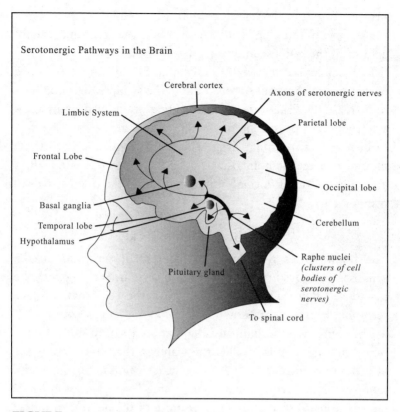

Serotonergic Pathways in the Brain

Cerebral cortex

Axons of serotonergic nerves

Limbic System

Parietal lobe

Frontal Lobe

Occipital lobe

Basal ganglia

Temporal lobe

Cerebellum

Hypothalamus

Raphe nuclei
(clusters of cell bodies of serotonergic nerves)

Pituitary gland

To spinal cord

FIGURE 2.2

about how the SSRIs disrupt the Serotonin. It is infinitely easier to figure out how something gets broken than to figure out how it actually works. Without identifying it as breakage, the drug companies have spent large amounts of money to study how the SSRIs initially impact the brain.

Imagine a conveyer belt that brings coal out of a mineshaft. If the conveyer becomes loaded down with other kinds of rocks, the coal won't fit onto the belt. As a result, the coal will collect at the bottom of the conveyer belt.

There is a chemical conveyor belt (or transporter system) that carries excess or unused serotonin from the synapse back into the neurons of origin. Prozac leaps onto the chemical conveyer belt for serotonin and clogs it up. As a result, the serotonin cannot get out of the synapse and instead remains behind.

By blocking the removal of serotonin, Eli Lilly and Co. hoped to increase the amount of serotonin in the synapse. The goal was to increase the firing rate of neurons that are influenced by serotonin. But it's not that simple, because the brain resists the effect of Prozac or any similar drug. The brain wants to return to its natural balance or homeostasis. The drug effect is, after all, a gross disruption of normal brain function, so the brain strives to overcome it.

The Brain Fights Back

The brain senses the abnormal increase of serotonin in the synapses and tries in several ways to reverse it. Starting with the first dose of Prozac or any other SSRI, the cells that produce serotonin begin to shut down. They stop releasing serotonin.

The shutdown mechanism is similar to a safety shutoff on a pump that fills a pool. When the water in the pool exceeds the safe or required depth, the rising water sends a signal to the pump to shut down. Similarly, the rising level of serotonin signals neurons to stop releasing any more of the neurotransmitter into the synapse.[7]

Early studies showed that this defense mechanism breaks down after a period of about ten days and the cells resume producing and releasing serotonin. However, there is evidence that the mechanism can continue to operate indefinitely in some areas of the brain.

In addition to shutting down the output of serotonin, the brain also compensates by becoming less sensitive to the effects of serotonin. When the brain senses that Prozac has caused too much serotonin to pool in the synapse, the brain reacts defensively by destroying its own receptors for serotonin. The receptors actually die back and disappear. In some regions of the brain, the dieback may result in losses of 40–60 percent of serotonin receptors.[8] The result of this well-known defensive mechanism is called subsensitivity or downregulation.

What is the overall outcome of this competition between the drug effect and the brain's attempt to overcome it? No one knows. As yet, there are no instruments or methods that can measure the concentration of serotonin or other chemical messengers in the synapses. We cannot measure the outcome of the struggle between Prozac and the brain's defense mechanisms.

Although there is no way to tell how much serotonin exists in any particular synapse, by grinding up an animal's brain it is possible to measure the overall amount of serotonin in the brain. Contrary to the original expectation, animal studies show that Prozac and other SSRIs do not increase the overall amount of serotonin bathing the cells in the whole brain. The failure of the SSRIs to increase overall brain serotonin may be due to the strength of the brain's compensatory mechanisms.

Yet another compensatory mechanism has been described. Remember that Prozac clogs the chemical transporter system that removes serotonin from the synapses between the neurons. A 1999 study by a team of scientists from Germany and the United States led by Viola Wegerer has now shown that the transporter system increases in density (there is a proliferation of transporters) after young rats have been exposed to Prozac for only two weeks. Thus, when the SSRIs clog the transport system, the transport system in turn fights back by becoming more dense, enabling it to continue removing serotonin from the synapses.

Unfortunately, the brain's compensatory changes can in themselves become a source of persistent or lifelong dysfunction. When that happens, the individual's brain becomes permanently abnormal.

Evidence for Permanent Damage and Dysfunction from SSRIs

In the Wegerer study, the increased transporter density persisted for at least ninety days into the adulthood of the rats. Furthermore, these seemingly permanent abnormalities were found in the most highly developed portion of the brain—the frontal lobes. The authors warn that administering SSRI antidepressants to children and youth during the periods of greatest brain development may result in lasting brain dysfunction.[9]

As the highest evolutionary development of the human being, the frontal lobes fill up the front of the skull, giving us our distinctive bulging forehead compared with the relatively flat-headed apes. When the frontal lobes are damaged, the human being is diminished in regard to his or her most human attributes, including judgment, conscience, self-understanding, and love.[10] It is especially ominous, therefore, that young animals develop permanent changes in the frontal lobes of their brains after a brief exposure to Prozac. Wegerer and her colleagues are to be commended for correctly pointing out that their data speaks to the danger of giving SSRIs to children. It also indicates a potential danger to adults, since the brain retains its reactivity to drugs as long as it is alive.

More Evidence for SSRI-Induced Brain Damage

The thalamus is a nerve center deeper in the brain that is richly interconnected with the frontal lobes. Old-fashioned lobotomies aimed at disrupting these connections. A research team from the Wayne State University School of Medicine studied children with obsessive-compulsive disorder before and after they took Paxil. The SSRI antidepressant caused shrinkage of brain tissue (loss of brain tissue) in the area of the thalamus. Unfortunately, these authors argue without justification in their May 2000 publication that the shrinkage may be good for the children.[11]

In a study by Yale University researchers published in December 2000, Prozac given to rats for two to four weeks stimulated an abnormal proliferation or increase in the number of neurons in a portion of the temporal lobe.[12] Remember that the Wayne State scientists argued that shrinkage (cell death) was good for patients. In sharp contrast, the Yale researchers argued in their report and in a press release that abnormal brain cell proliferation might be good for patients. When drug advocates discover that their drugs are damaging the brains of animals or humans, they tend to justify it on the grounds that the damage was caused by the patient's mental illness or that it was good for the patients. Seldom do they openly admit that their drugs harm the brain.

The rationalization offered by the Yale researchers was especially bizarre. As evidence that the drug-induced brain damage might be helpful to patients, they pointed out that shock treatment also causes abnormal cell proliferation in the temporal lobe. They didn't stop to realize that shock treatment causes permanent memory loss and damage to other mental functions precisely because of its traumatic impact on the temporal lobes.

Yet another study of Prozac effects on rat brain function found grossly reduced cerebral metabolism as measured by the brain's use of glucose.[13] The average reductions in two regions reached 23 percent and 32 percent. In other words, the brain's overall metabolic rate (its rate of energy utilization and hence its overall function) was substantially compromised.

Consistent with the widespread nature of the serotonin nerve network, changes were found throughout the brain, including the highest centers of the brain in the cerebral cortex (surface) and the movement centers in the basal ganglia (deeper in the brain). The widespread nature of these harmful effects help accounts for the varied nature of adverse effects produced by Prozac. However, the authors, as drug advocates, conclude that these gross reductions in function throughout the brain might be the source of a "therapeutic" effect.

Brain cell death, abnormal brain cell growth—either one can be rationalized as therapeutic by advocates of biological psychiatry and drugs. This kind of bizarre rationalization of drug-induced brain damage is commonplace in psychiatry but is not generally accepted in other fields of medicine where drug-induced damage is usually recognized for what it is.

Meanwhile, the evidence is piling up that SSRIs cause permanent brain damage. A study in *Brain Research* has shown that single doses of Prozac and Luvox, as well as desipramine, caused abnormal growth in brain cells in the temporal region in young rats.[14] The abnormalities persisted at the time of the last examination three weeks after treatment. The authors concluded that these results "raise the possibility that chronic fluoxetine [Prozac] treatment arrests [nerve cell] development into young adulthood."

Another recent study in *Brain Research* has found that four days of high doses of Prozac and Zoloft, as well as other serotonin-stimulating drugs, caused marked changes in brain cells, including the bodies of the cells and projections called axons.[15] Prozac most commonly produced a "large swelling" in the body of neurons. Zoloft produced "swollen and truncated" axons and in some cases made the neurons "corkscrew" in shape. The study voices concern about whether these injured cells could survive, but leaves the question unanswered. The authors suggest this damage could indicate the long-term effect of chronic SSRI use.

Drug Company Responses to the Danger of Permanent Damage

Although drug companies have spent millions of dollars demonstrating the acute or immediate effects of their antidepressant drugs on the brain, they have spent almost nothing on the most important question—"Does the brain *ever* recover from these effects?" Keep in mind that the brain's receptors for serotonin die back after being exposed to SSRI drugs. Anyone taking these drugs should want to know if their brain receptors ever grow back. If not, then their brain will remain chronically impaired with a reduced level of reactivity in the serotonin system.

It would be reassuring to believe that the brain will recover from the dysfunction and damage caused by the antidepressants, but scientists know from the example of other medications that this is not necessarily so. The class of drugs called antipsychotics or neuroleptics, for example, commonly produces permanent damage to the brain. This became recognized only because the damage results in obvious twitches, spasms, and other abnormal movements that cannot be ignored.

It also has been known for some time that drugs with similar chemical effects to the SSRI antidepressants can cause permanent damage to the brain's serotonin system. For example, the stimulants amphetamine and methamphetamine overstimulate serotonin in a somewhat similar fashion to antidepressants, and they are proven to cause permanent dysfunction in the serotonin system. They can even kill serotonin brain cells.

Meanwhile, it would not be difficult to conduct a series of basic experiments that determine, once and for all, the degree of danger to the brain posed by SSRIs. The first part of the necessary study has been done many times already in labs around the world. In these experiments, animals are treated with Prozac or another SSRI for several days or weeks. Then their brains are ground up and chemically analyzed to measure the amount and density of their serotonin receptors. That's how researchers quickly discovered that a large percentage of some classes of serotonin receptors begin to die back shortly after the animal is given its first dose of Prozac.

Only one more step is required to find out if the brain can recover from receptor dieback caused by Prozac or any other SSRI. After stopping the Prozac, some of the animals could be kept alive for a few more weeks or months. Then their brains could be studied to see if the receptors had recovered to normal levels. Other methods involving the use of brain scans with radioactive tracers can be used in living animals to determine the density of receptors. Both methods have been used in the studies previously cited in this chapter as indicating potentially permanent damage.

Looking for the Critical Research

When I first realized the implications of receptor loss and other brain malfunctions caused by SSRIs, I searched the literature looking for studies aimed at determining if the brain can recover.

I found numerous studies confirming the acute damage caused by the drugs, but no studies—until the recently published ones—that attempted to measure any potential recovery.

When I became the medical expert in charge of investigating the scientific basis for the first series of product liability lawsuits surrounding Prozac-induced murder and suicide (described in the introduction and in Chapter 15), I was able to frame questions to be asked of Eli Lilly and Co. executives and researchers. Under my direction, lawyers asked the head of research at Eli Lilly and Co., Dr. Ray Fuller, if the company had conducted any research concerning the brain's ability to recover from Prozac. Dr. Fuller admitted that as of 1994 no such research had been done by the company. Furthermore, he was unaware of anyone else conducting such research. When pressed to justify the company's failure to find out if the brain can recover from Prozac-induced changes, including the death of serotonin receptors, Fuller replied under oath, "I don't see that that would be of any value to know that."[16]

Unfortunately, it's readily apparent why a drug company would avoid conducting or publishing research concerning the ability of the brain to recover from its drug. The company seems reluctant to support research that might interfere with the mammoth profits generated by Prozac sales. Eli Lilly and Co. has a history of avoiding and even suppressing research that might cast doubt on the safety of Prozac (see the introduction and later chapters). I asked a prominent researcher in the field of receptor research why he didn't conduct a recovery study. He replied that it could "hurt Eli Lilly in court." He openly admitted that he received grants from the drug company. Another researcher told me he wouldn't even dare raise these issues in his pharmacology laboratory.

Without actual studies of the animal brain, there's no way to determine if people are recovering from taking these drugs. Subtle changes in mental function, such as memory or concentration difficulties or emotional blunting, are especially difficult to measure. It becomes difficult to determine if they are caused by a physical trauma, such as psychiatric drug exposure, or if they are caused by emotional problems. Since serotonin nerves spread throughout the brain, it's also difficult to anticipate how permanent damage would manifest itself in the life of the individual. It could affect not only mental function, but hormonal balances and a variety of other bodily functions. In addition, the person who has been harmed by a drug is often the last one to perceive the damage. In my clinical experience, people can be reduced to robotic, nearly stuporous states by drugs without appreciating what has happened to them. Often their families are the first to notice the growing mental incapacity and become concerned enough to tell the doctor.

Meanwhile, research confirms the concerns I raised for many years. Studies are showing dramatic and sometimes permanent changes in the brains of animals treated with SSRI antidepressants. It is time to mount a national research effort to study the problem.

Anticipating the Nature of Permanent Dysfunction

Despite the difficulty in predicting how permanent damage would manifest itself in the life of the individual, we can make some tentative predictions. Very probably, it would resemble a prolonged withdrawal reaction. In other words, the brain would go into withdrawal and then not recover. Most commonly, withdrawal symptoms manifest as the opposite effect from the drug. So a prolonged or even persistent withdrawal can include feelings of depression, numbness, anxiety, or irritability. It can involve odd, distressing "electrical" feelings in the brain or headaches. Some people "crash" and remain tired all the time. People who have lost weight while taking Prozac can end up gaining weight and becoming obese. A smaller number of people

develop permanent twitches or spasms. I will examine withdrawal effects in greater detail later in the book.

We Know Enough to Be Concerned

Prozac, Zoloft, Paxil, Celexa, and Luvox—SSRI antidepressants—disrupt the serotonin system of the brain by blocking the
removal of serotonin from the synapses. The intention is to acti-
vate the firing of the serotonin nerve cells—to put them into
overdrive. But the brain fights back against the Prozac effect, and
no one knows the net effect or overall outcome. It is not known
if there is a sustained increase in serotonin in any of the synapses.

Although drug companies have documented the existence of
dramatic SSRI-induced malfunctions in the brain, they have
avoided research concerning the brain's potential to recover.
However, a flurry of recently published independent research has
confirmed concerns that I first expressed several years ago—that
the drug-induced brain changes are in fact drastic and probably
can become permanent.

Meanwhile, science has almost no understanding of how the
widespread serotonin system functions in the brain. Basically, we
don't know what it does. We only know that we are disrupting
and damaging it with SSRIs.

In a frightening but realistic sense, taking Prozac or other
SSRIs is like a stab in the dark—a chemical thrust into the largely
unexplored, unmapped region of life that is your brain.

THREE

Dangerously Stimulating the Brain and Mind with Antidepressants[1]

Jane had never been "mentally ill" in her life. She took the SSRI antidepressant because she felt a little "blue" and her family doctor thought it might help. After about a month on the antidepressant, Jane began to feel "wonderful—better than ever." She needed less sleep, had more energy, lost as much weight as she wanted, and got a lot done at home and at work. At first, friends and family alike were grateful for the changes in her.

Then one day Jane went out and bought a car with cash. This by itself might not have seemed excessive or irrational, except the family was already paying off loans on two other cars that were in fine working condition, and the money that she spent was needed to pay their taxes. Jane brushed off her husband's complaints.

Now Jane seemed to need hardly any sleep at all. She was becoming, in her own words, "a lean, mean fighting machine." Her mind was always going "a mile a minute" and she loved the feeling of being "charged up." When her husband continued to express worry about her excessive spending and her increasingly angry and unpredictable moods, she moved out and left him to take care of the home and the children.

Jane's family doctor now became concerned about her seemingly unstable emotions. Believing that she was becoming "mentally ill," he referred her to a psychiatrist.

Jane's husband loved her very much and feared that the antidepressant was causing her behavior to deteriorate. When he called her new psychiatrist to express his concern, he was "blown off" by him. Because it had initially seemed to help her, the psychiatrist actually increased Jane's SSRI antidepressant dose and added a "mood stabilizer" to "slow her down a bit."

At work Jane became increasingly resentful at her boss's failure to accept her plans for the future of the company. He explained she wasn't even supposed to be involved in that arena. After having several temper tantrums, she was fired.

Two days later, Jane was picked up by the police for causing an altercation in a supermarket with a clerk who wasn't "treating her with enough respect." Jane had cut ahead of everyone else in the line and was threatening physical violence against the clerk and the store manager when the police arrived. The police could see that she was "mentally ill" and took her against her will to an emergency room. She was admitted involuntarily to the hospital's psychiatric unit.

In the hospital doctors wanted to start Jane on antipsychotic drugs—while keeping her on the original SSRI antidepressant and the mood stabilizer. Her husband, who still loved and cared for her, tried to intervene. Jane, fortunately, told the doctors she wanted to go home with her husband. After legal threats by her husband, the hospital discharged Jane with the proviso that she continue taking all of her medications.

At home, Jane and her husband sought a second opinion. The new doctor diagnosed Jane as suffering from a classic case of SSRI-induced mania. He explained that the antidepressant drug reaction was well known and should have been recognized by the various doctors who had seen and treated her. He began the process of withdrawing her from all medication and helping her to heal the wounds she had created in her family.

Over several months Jane became herself again. But she remained traumatized by the consequences of her behavior, including the harm she did to her family and her career, her arrest record, and her incarceration in a mental hospital. She is suing the doctor and the drug company but no amount of money will fully compensate her.

No Scientific Doubt

It is understandable if the lay reader shows skepticism toward the idea that routinely used antidepressants can make people like Jane suffer from mania and psychosis so that they end up ruining their lives. But no one familiar with drug effects should question the scientific conclusion that all antidepressants can cause mania.

The *Diagnostic and Statistical Manual of Mental Disorders, IV* (1994), published by the American Psychiatric Association, is the most commonly used source of diagnostic information in the field of mental health. It provides the source of official diagnoses for insurance company reimbursement, FDA drug approval studies, and most research projects in the field. It is also commonly cited in court.

Both before and after the development of SSRI antidepressants, the manual has consistently confirmed that all antidepressants can cause mania. The most recent edition states, for example, "Symptoms like those seen in a Manic Episode may also be precipitated by antidepressant treatment such as medication. . . . "[2] The manual repeats this observation on several other occasions as well.

All of the SSRIs

Jane's story is a composite of many cases I have seen and researched involving all of the SSRI antidepressants. Right now I'm involved as a medical consultant in a product liability case against Eli Lilly and Co. concerning a doctor who became manic while taking Prozac. His career was completely ruined by his irrational violent actions while taking the drug.

I am also a treating physician or consultant for several other patients who became manic when they were taking Prozac and other SSRIs. For most purposes, SSRI drugs can be considered the same in regard to their overall effects, including their tendency to cause mania.

Mania is a form of extreme overstimulation. All of the SSRIs can cause stimulation in the form of insomnia, anxiety, agitation, and nervousness. Although some clinicians believe that Zoloft, for example, has a less stimulating effect, all SSRIs are frequently stimulating, and all can sometimes be sedating.

The FDA clinical studies for Zoloft, Paxil, and Celexa reported higher rates of sexual dysfunction than the clinical studies for Prozac. Differences like this may be due to different reporting criteria or to the growing awareness among clinicians that SSRIs commonly cause sexual dysfunction. *In general, if one SSRI produces a particular adverse effect, the others probably will do so as well. Many textbooks discuss Prozac, Zoloft, Paxil, Celexa, and Zoloft as a group without mentioning many differences. The main differences, such as the intensity of acute withdrawal symptoms, will be discussed as we go along.*

The Stimulant Profile

Stimulation can manifest itself in many ways, including insomnia, increased energy, agitation, anxiety, nervousness, tremors, loss of appetite, and weight loss. These effects are the same as those caused by the classic stimulants—methylphenidate (Ritalin), amphetamine, methamphetamine, Ecstasy, and cocaine.

There's a biochemical explanation for the similar effects between the SSRIs and the classic stimulants. Both groups of drugs rev up the serotonin system in the brain. The stimulants, however, jack up two additional chemical messengers, dopamine and nor-epinephrine, probably accounting for their even greater tendency to cause overstimulation.

The similarities between the SSRIs and the stimulants show up during withdrawal as well. When you try to stop taking SSRIs, you can suffer an emotionally distressing withdrawal that includes "crashing" with depression, fatigue, and feelings of hopelessness. This is similar to the amphetamines and cocaine. But withdrawal from the SSRIs can be much more difficult than withdrawal from amphetamines. SSRI withdrawal commonly involves painful physical symptoms, such as a flulike syndrome, muscle cramps, and shock-like headaches.

Despite similarities in regard to withdrawal responses, SSRI antidepressants do not commonly produce the kind of dependence characteristic of stimulants. There are relatively few reports of individuals becoming hooked on ever-increasing doses of SSRIs. This is partly because the SSRIs tend, if anything, to cause more distressing adverse effects as the doses are escalated, without continuing to produce the kind of euphoria or artificial sense of well-being associated with the stimulants.

However, people can find it very difficult to stop taking SSRIs, and like amphetamine addicts, they can end up desperately in need of continuing the SSRIs to stave off withdrawal symptoms. In the *International Journal of Risk and Safety in Medicine*, I reported on the case of a young woman who "crashed" and became desperate when she ran out of her Prozac while away from home.

Causing Mania

The stimulating effects of SSRIs are demonstrated by what happens when people like Jane have more extreme or exaggerated reactions to the drugs. Mania—a potentially psychotic condition of intense mental and emotional excitement—is the most extreme manifestation of SSRI-induced stimulation. Mania is often accompanied by feelings of Godlike power, invulnerability, racing thoughts, unrealistic elaborate plans, and violence.

In my practice and as a medical expert, I've evaluated people like Jane whose lives have been ruined as a result of SSRI-caused mania. They have broken with loved ones, wasted their savings, robbed banks or committed violence. Their actions have been obviously self-destructive or doomed to failure, and totally incompatible with their character and conduct prior to ever taking an SSRI. The next two chapters will deal with suicide and then violence under the influence of SSRIs. These actions often take place during mania or after collapse into its opposite, depression.

SSRI-induced mania is not rare. It is, in fact, common. The FDA found that Prozac caused mania in a little more than 1 percent of depressed patients. The rate would be much higher in clinical practice where patients aren't being observed once a week by highly experienced investigators. The FDA defines 1 percent—one in 100 persons—as common. The occurrence of mania in 1 out of 100 people during short clinical trials represents a significant public health danger.

A recent controlled clinical trial of Prozac in children disclosed a striking 6 percent rate of mania. This was so disconcerting to the prodrug researchers that they hid the data in a section about causes for dropouts and didn't comment on it in the abstract, discussion, or summary.[3]

When patients become manic on antidepressants, doctors commonly tell their patients that the mania "emerged" during the drug treatment, as if the mania were there to begin with, and was merely "triggered" or "brought out" by the drug. We know that this isn't true in regard to Prozac. We know, instead, that Prozac can cause mania in people who have never shown any manic tendencies.

In reviewing all of the reported cases of mania during the clinical trials used to approve Prozac, the FDA found that the new antidepressant was nearly four times more likely to cause mania than the older antidepressant given to the same patients. Mania occurred in 1.1 percent of the Prozac-treated patients compared with 0.3 percent of patients given amitriptyline (Elavil). Seventy percent of the patients who became manic on Prozac had never shown any signs of manic tendencies in the past. By contrast, all of the patients who became manic on the older antidepressant turned out to have had a past history of mania.[4]

These scientific findings confirm that Prozac, perhaps unlike older antidepressants, commonly causes mania in patients who otherwise have no potential in that direction. However, Eli Lilly and Co. never made this data public and, unless they have read my books, practicing physicians have no idea about it. The all-important data was kept off the label for Prozac and the drug company never made it known to the profession. I found the data when reviewing the FDA files for my forensic work. But even if SSRIs only "brought out" an underlying mania, the drugs are nonetheless drastically worsening the patient's condition.

A rate of a little more than 1 percent for mania may not immediately strike the reader as very high. But imagine a room filled with 100 people. Now imagine that, like clockwork, one of these people will become manic, and probably psychotic, after the entire group has taken Prozac for only a few weeks.

Also keep in mind that mania is a very destructive disorder that includes wildly out-of-control behavior, a loss of impulse control, extreme actions like spending a life savings in a matter of days, and sometimes criminal activities and violence. Also keep in mind, as I will emphasize throughout this book, that the rate will be far higher in actual practice than in the clinical trials. Clinical trials are very short (averaging four or five weeks for Prozac), much more carefully monitored than clinical practice, and comparatively selective in who gets treated. If the rate of mania is about 1 percent under these conditions, it will inevitably be several times higher under real-world conditions where patients have more complicated and often more severe problems, where they will receive the drug for months and years at a time, and where doctors often lack knowledge or ability to supervise the patient on a weekly basis. However, even at a conservatively estimated rate of 1 percent, 10 out of every 1,000 patients will become manic on SSRIs.

All of the SSRIs can cause mania. The drug-induced disorder occurred in approximately 1 percent of patients given Paxil for depression during the FDA trials. That was more than three times the rate at which mania appeared in the same or similar group of depressed patients taking placebo. Therefore the Paxil, rather than preexisting depression or a latent tendency to mania, was the cause of the mania.

Mania in response to Luvox occurred in a whopping 4 percent of depressed youngsters (ages eight–seventeen) during the FDA trials, whereas it never occurred in the control group of similar young patients who were administered placebo.

If government agencies or organized psychiatry were sufficiently concerned about SSRI-induced mania and psychosis, they could carry out additional epidemiological studies to evaluate its frequency and severity. These have not been conducted. However, psychiatrist Malcolm B. Bowers Jr. from Yale University told a reporter that their research found that "SSRI-induced psychosis has accounted for 8% of all general hospital psychiatric admissions over a recent 14-month period."[5]

Burying the Mania Threat

Although the original label for Prozac did not deal with the special danger of Prozac causing mania in patients with no history of mania, it did at least make clear in the PRECAUTIONS section that the rate was approximately 1 percent: "During premarketing testing, hypomania or mania occurred in approximately 1% of fluoxetine-treated patients." These observations remained unchanged for many years through the 1997 label.

However, in 1998 the drug company convinced the FDA to accept a greatly modified discussion of Prozac-induced mania, apparently based on a hodgepodge of clinical trials carried out before and after drug approval. One can be sure that the FDA didn't check on the validity of all those trials. It doesn't have the manpower or the commitment. From now on, the mania section of the label would begin with the following observation: "In US placebo-controlled clinical trials for depression, mania/hypomania was reported in 0.1% of patients treated with Prozac and 0.1% of patients treated with placebo."

According to this new "improved" data, Prozac doesn't cause mania at all in depressed patients, or at least no more frequently than a sugar pill. That, of course, is scientifically unsound and contradicts the body of scientific research in the public domain. The data is also meaningless, since we don't know how many patients were involved in the various groups, how long the studies were, under what rules they were conducted, and who supervised and sponsored them.

The paragraph then explains that the rate of mania/hypomania in controlled clinical trials for obsessive-compulsive disorder was 0.8 percent—eight times higher than the rates for people who are depressed. This, of course, makes no clinical sense at all. Depression is far more likely to be associated with mania (hence the term, manic-depressive disorder) than is obsessive-compulsive disorder.

To add to the confusion, the paragraph about mania concludes with the following statement: "In all US Prozac clinical trials, 0.7% of 10,782 patients reported mania/hypomania." What is the difference between the source of the 0.1 percent rate and 0.7 percent rate? Apparently, the higher rate includes clinical trials that were not placebo-controlled.

The data in this new paragraph in the Prozac label is no longer taken from FDA psychiatrist Richard Kapit's analysis of the more carefully monitored controlled clinical trials used for FDA approval of the drug. Instead, the company has been allowed to use their own analysis of an unspecified number of U.S. clinical trials most or all of which apparently took place after the marketing of the drug. Pooling varied studies using different rules and investigators is epidemiologically unsound. Unlike the FDA trials, which

I was able to evaluate and to largely debunk in *Talking Back to Prozac,* this pooled data remains unavailable for critical examination. If the pooling of these unspecified clinical trials did in fact result in this kind of nonsense, then the process was undoubtedly badly flawed and invalid.

The changes in the 1998 Prozac label that obscure the danger of drug-induced mania exemplify the marketing genius of Eli Lilly and Co. Initially forced to put a simple warning in the label about a 1 percent risk of mania in depressed patients taking Prozac, they have bamboozled the FDA into accepting a confusing, misleading, self-contradictory, and hard to decipher paragraph that totally obscures the problem for the busy physician who tries to read the label.

Overall, harmful degrees of stimulation are a much more common SSRI effect than most doctors appreciate. Unfortunately, doctors often mistake the drug-induced agitation and anxiety for an "anxiety disorder" within the patient, and they end up prescribing sedative or tranquilizing drugs like Klonopin, Xanax, Ativan, or Valium. Instead, they should stop the SSRI.

Hiding the Truth from the Beginning

It should have been obvious from the beginning that Prozac and all other SSRIs would cause stimulation and mania. In fact, it should have been clear that Prozac posed the whole range of dangers found with stimulants like amphetamine, methamphetamine, and cocaine.

Indeed, Eli Lilly and Co. found out about Prozac's stimulating effects long before the drug went to market. They discovered the problem early in their clinical trials. During the approval process, the FDA, as well as British, German, and French agencies, raised serious questions about the stimulating effect.

The BGA, the German equivalent of the FDA, was so concerned about the stimulating effects of Prozac that it asked the drug company to conduct a study of its clinical trials to determine how many patients were overstimulated. Charles Beasley, an executive in Eli Lilly and Co.'s Division of Neurosciences, compiled a secret report, "Activation and Sedation in Fluoxetine Clinical Studies." Beasley counted the cases in which patients displayed "nervousness, anxiety, agitation, insomnia." Beasley found that a whopping 38 percent of Prozac patients were afflicted with these adverse effects during the short clinical trials. The percentage would have been even higher if he had included other obvious signs of stimulation, such as hyperactivity, euphoria, and mania.

His results were so damaging to Prozac that the report was never released to the German agency, to the FDA, or to anyone else. Eli Lilly and Co. hid the data. I found the report in the company files when I was reviewing materials for product liability suits against the drug company and subsequently testified about it in court.

Patients were getting so overstimulated that a large portion of them were dropping out of the Prozac trials, causing the Prozac trials to fail. If a drug is so harmful that many or most patients stop taking it, the drug is not likely to get FDA approval. Also, most doctors are aware that stimulating drugs can be dangerous. The drug company wanted to avoid giving Prozac a reputation for stimulating patients.

Deciding to Cover Up the Stimulating Effects

Patients were getting so overstimulated from the start of the clinical trials for FDA approval that Eli Lilly's top scientist, Ray Fuller, issued the following in-house secret order: "Some patients have converted from severe depression to agitation within a few days [of starting Prozac]. In one case the agitation was marked and the patient had to be taken off the drug. In future studies, the use of benzodiazepines [tranquilizers] to control agitation will be permitted."

Fuller's secret order to give benzodiazepine tranquilizers like Valium, Klonopin, and Xanax broke the rules. The FDA-approved rules for the clinical trials prohibited the use of tranquilizers along with Prozac. Giving the tranquilizers made it impossible to tell the difference between Prozac effects and tranquilizer effects. It also exposed the patients to dangerous, addictive tranquilizers like Klonopin, Xanax, and Valium that are only supposed to be used for a few weeks at a time. Finally, it partially covered up Prozac's dangerous tendency to cause stimulation. Yet despite these attempts to minimize the stimulating effect, a great deal of evidence surfaced indicating that Prozac was dangerously stimulating for many if not most patients.

After several years the FDA began to catch on to the trick of giving the Prozac patients tranquilizers to try to calm them down. By now the drug company had invested millions of dollars in the drug. It also had powerful connections in the government. President George Bush had been on the board of directors of Eli Lilly and Co. Vice President Dan Quayle was from Indiana, the home state of Eli Lilly and Co., and had former company employees on his staff.

When the FDA realized what Eli Lilly and Co. had done, it must have seemed too late to do anything about it. Nonetheless, in regard to one of the key clinical trials used for approval of the drug, the FDA demanded an accounting of the patients who had been put on tranquilizers against the rules. At the same time, it became apparent that Prozac could not be approved as effective if the tranquilized patients were not included. The multimillion-dollar trials were turning out to be an utter failure—a financial catastrophe for the drug company that had spent multimillions on the drug and was banking on it to rescue the company. So the FDA decided to rescue the pharmaceutical company. Patients who took a combination of Prozac and addictive tranquilizers were included in the final evaluation of Prozac's effectiveness, and as a result, Prozac squeaked through. With a lot of statistical manipulation, Prozac plus tranquilizers came out marginally effective, and the FDA approved the drug.

Thus the FDA approved Prozac in combination with addictive tranquilizers, but the medical profession and the public were never informed until I documented this sordid affair in great detail in *Talking Back to Prozac.*

Dissent Within the FDA

Meanwhile, not everyone at the FDA was happy with this surrender to the political interests of the administration and the drug company. Richard Kapit, the FDA psychiatrist in charge of evaluating the safety of Prozac, repeatedly warned his superiors that Prozac was dangerously similar to stimulants like amphetamine and cocaine.

In several internal FDA memos, Kapit warned that Prozac "resembles the profile of a stimulant . . ." He specifically compared Prozac to amphetamine. He was concerned that Prozac's tendency to cause "insomnia, nervousness, anorexia, and weight loss" could actually worsen depression in some patients. He wanted Eli Lilly and Co. to rewrite the label so that Prozac's stimulating effects would be more obvious to doctors. He also raised these issues in the FDA hearing that is routinely held before the approval of new drugs for marketing. Kapit came to these conclusions without having the benefit of reviewing the concerns being raised at the European agencies, and without the benefit of the secret in-house Eli Lilly and Co. report on activation caused by Prozac.

Nothing came of Kapit's concerns. Kapit's boss, Paul Leber, rejected his warnings. Leber, as I mentioned in the introduction, is now working as a consultant to drug companies.

Are other SSRI antidepressants as stimulating as Prozac? Based on my findings about Zoloft that I obtained through freedom of information from the FDA. The data confirms that "Agitation" and "insomnia" were among the common reasons patients stopped taking the drug, and that tranquilizing drugs were often given to calm down the patients.

Although the Germans never received important hidden data from Eli Lilly and Co., they remained concerned enough to put a special warning in the German label for the drug. The German label for Prozac warns that patients should be given tranquilizers early in their treatment to counteract stimulation and to prevent suicide.

Summing Up the Stimulant Pattern

Meanwhile, a careful reading of the Prozac label as found in the 2001 *Physicians' Desk Reference* does disclose the stimulant pattern. Not all of the following adverse effects are specific for stimulation, but they are related to it and can be caused by classical stimulants like methylphenidate (Ritalin), amphetamine, methamphetamine, and cocaine. Based on reports from Prozac clinical trials as summarized in the 2001 label, here is a compilation of *psychiatric adverse effects* that are *frequently* (occuring in at least 1 percent) caused by Prozac:[6]

Insomnia (16–33 percent)
Sleep disorder (frequent)
Abnormal dreams (1–5 percent)
Somnolence (13–17 percent)
Nervousness (11–14 percent)
Agitation (frequent)
Anxiety (12–15 percent)
Tremor (10 percent)
Hypomania and mania (over 1 percent in depression trials)
Emotional lability [instability] (frequent)
Confusion (frequent)
Dizziness (10 percent)
Amnesia (frequent)
Libido decreased (3–11 percent)

A number of other drug-induced psychiatric problems are mentioned in the label as *infrequently* reported during the clinical trials. All of them are also caused by stimulant drugs:

Acute brain syndrome (global mental dysfunction)
Akathisia (a form of agitation)
Apathy
Central nervous system depression
Central nervous system stimulation
Depersonalization
Euphoria
Hallucinations
Hostility
Paranoid reaction
Personality disorder
Psychosis

In addition, a number of gastrointestinal and other symptoms associated with Prozac are also typical of stimulant drugs. The most important and closely related to stimulation are anorexia and weight loss. All of the classic stimulants from Ritalin to cocaine also cause anorexia and weight loss. A further discussion of gastrointestinal and bodily adverse drug effects will be found in Chapter 4.

The above compilation of adverse stimulantlike effects indicates a serious problem with these drugs that should discourage doctors and patients alike. Although based on the drug company's tainted data collection and analysis, it nonetheless paints a threatening picture of the potential dangers to the brain and mind associated with taking Prozac (and other SSRIs). However, the data is spread out in several different places in the label, and required my painstaking compilation to fully present the size of the problem. Overall, probably about one-half or more of patients taking Prozac develop stimulant symptoms of one kind or another. Remember, the drug company's own internal analysis showed that 38 percent of patients in short controlled clinical trials developed signs of stimulation, and its report did not consider all the possible signs of stimulation. Also remember that many of these patients were taking tranquilizers to calm them down and to hide their symptoms of stimulation.

The Insidious Danger of Akathisia

Furthermore, the SSRIs commonly cause another stimulantlike effect that can lead to dangerous behavior. It is called akathisia. Akathisia was also left out of consideration in Beasley's analysis of how many patients became stimulated.

Akathisia is a neurological disorder that is commonly caused by all of the SSRIs. Akathisia means the inability to sit or stand still. It can feel as if someone is dragging chalk down a blackboard, only it's inside your brain and down your spinal cord. Akathisia is a dreadful feeling that compels the victim to keep moving in an effort to relieve it.

Akathisia is listed as "infrequent" on the Prozac label. Actually, Eli Lilly and Co. systematically avoided looking for akathisia in the clinical trials. In later, more independent studies, akathisia turned out to be very common. As I documented in my medical textbook, *Brain-Disabling Treatments in Psychiatry* (1997), reported rates of akathisia from taking Prozac range from 10 to 25 percent.[7] In Chapters 6 and 7 I shall examine how akathisia can drive people to suicide and violence.

Although doctors are becoming more aware that the SSRIs can cause akathisia, they too frequently miss the diagnosis. They often mistake akathisia for their patients "getting anxious" or "agitated," and so they mistakenly increase the SSRI dosage, worsening the condition of their patients. Eventually these doctors add new drugs to deal with the "anxiety." As a result, many patients end up taking increasing doses and numbers of drugs that aggravate and complicate their original problems with new drug-induced disorders. In my psychiatric practice, I often find that patients improve as their drugs are gradually removed one by one. They are shocked but gratified to find themselves much better off without any drugs.

Doctors remain misinformed in part because they obtain too much of their information from drug company representatives and advertisements. The seemingly scientific workshops they attend are often little more than drug company–sponsored advertising sessions. Also, doctors often find it easier to blame a problem on the patient's "mental illness" rather than on the drugs that they have prescribed for them.

Since medication-impaired patients often have little or no idea what is happening to them, they cannot point to their drugs as the culprit. Doctors, in turn, often dismiss their patients' "complaints" as irrational or as due to their mental problems rather than to the drugs prescribed by the doctor. Also, many drug-induced adverse reactions seem bizarre. The experience of akathisia, for example, is so distressing and strange that patients sound irrational when attempting to describe it. They say things like "I have electricity going through my veins" or "It's like someone is scraping my nerves with a knife edge." Unfortunately, many doctors don't recognize these statements as typical descriptions of akathisia. They may even misdiagnose the patient as suffering from delusions or hallucinations, and add neuroleptic drugs like Risperdal or Haldol that commonly worsen akathisia.

Variability in Patient Reactions

The recognition of potential adverse drug effects is complicated by the variability of response among patients. For example, not everyone gets overstimulated by SSRIs. In fact, some patients experience the opposite. They become more sedated rather than stimulated. In the Prozac clinical trials for FDA approval, asthenia (weakness, malaise) was reported in 12 percent and somnolence in 13 percent of patients taking the drug. SSRIs also commonly make people feel lethargic, fatigued, tired, or "blah."

Sometimes the patient endures a confusing mixture of anxiety and sedation, a kind of agitated fatigue or depression.

Unfortunately, these drug reactions frequently get blamed on the patient's depression. Once again the drug dose is increased, or new drugs are added, instead of stopping the offending drug. Meanwhile, the patient's condition deteriorates, and that too is blamed on the individual's "mental illness" rather than on the mounting adverse drug effects.

When these patients come to me for a consultation as a doctor of last resort, they are far more depressed and despairing than they were months or years earlier at the start of their treatment. In my experience, doctors who prescribe psychiatric drugs expect many of their patients to get worse during treatment and they attribute it to the "natural course" of the depression or anxiety. I never start patients on antidepressants, and in my experience as a psychiatrist and psychotherapist, it is rare for patients to get worse during treatment. Indeed, I consider it a major treatment failure if this happens. In most cases, their depression begins to lift as they are safely withdrawn from the drugs and as they receive therapy to deal with their personal problems.

Other patients on Prozac report experiencing little or no effect of any kind, good or bad, from taking routine doses of SSRIs. Still others experience what they describe as good effects without any serious adverse ones. In later chapters, I will raise doubts about the nature of these seemingly "good" effects.

Overall, there is a wide range of reactions to the SSRIs. People can also react differently at different times or at varying doses or when doses are being raised or lowered or when other drugs are added or removed.

We don't know why some people react with stimulation and others with sedation to these drugs. However, we do know that some people have a genetic inability to adequately remove Prozac and other drugs from their body. Although most physicians don't realize it, this genetic difficulty in ridding the body of these drugs is very common. And there are tests to check for it. I will discuss this important problem in a separate chapter.

We have only begun to examine the harmful effects of the SSRI antidepressants. Remember that serotonin nerves spread through the brain and also impact the pituitary gland that controls the release of hormones that affect endocrine, stress, sexual, and growth processes. In addition, the chemical serotonin is found throughout the body, including in the platelets (blood clotting agents), in the bloodstream, and cells in the gut. Once again, the function of serotonin in these various parts of the body is not understood.

Overall, an immense variety of painful and harmful effects are caused by the SSRIs. But in my experience, three different kinds of effects are particularly harmful: (1) mania, psychosis, and other extreme mental and behavioral reactions; (2) sexual dysfunction; and (3) withdrawal problems when trying to stop the SSRIs.

This chapter has focused on stimulation and related adverse effects of SSRIs. The next chapter addresses the broader range of adverse effects caused by the SSRIs. Later chapters will examine the negative impact on behavior and personal relationships.

FOUR

Multiple Additional Risks When Taking SSRI Antidepressants

A woman takes Celexa and within weeks she loses interest in sex, even though she continues to love her husband. A man takes Prozac and notices that he's developing blue blotches under his skin as if he's bleeding too easily from minor bruises. Another woman takes Zoloft and soon has ringing in her ears. A man takes Paxil and becomes lethargic. Yet another takes Luvox and develops a disfiguring facial tic that will not go away even when the drug is stopped. A child takes Paxil and suddenly cannot sit still. He becomes a "hyperactive kid" for the first time. Another child develops palpitations of the heart on Prozac.

How can one distinct group of drugs, the SSRIs, cause so many varied adverse effects—especially when they are supposed to be so safe?

Lemonade out of Lemons

As one of the most profitable of all industries, the pharmaceutical industries are among the more competitive and even cutthroat. They must make ever-increasing profits to maintain the level of financial return demanded by investors. Toward that goal, drug companies mount sales campaigns to convince doctors and patients to use their new products rather than older, more familiar ones. The drug companies spend thousands of dollars every year influencing each doctor in the United States, and to influence potential patients as well. To do so effectively, the drug company needs a unique "sales pitch" tailored to their specific drug.

When clinical trials repeatedly showed that Prozac was not as effective as the older antidepressants, Eli Lilly and Co. developed an advertising campaign that proved successful beyond anyone's anticipation. The drug company played up the supposed safety of Prozac. This unjustified claim set the tone for the promotion of future SSRIs as well.

There is little or no basis to the claim of greater safety but there are differences in the kinds of adverse effects caused by the older antidepressants and the SSRIs. Most of the older so-called tricyclic antidepressants such as amitriptyline and doxepin tend to be sedating and to cause weight gain. The SSRIs tend to be more stimulating and, initially at least, to cause weight loss. It's like comparing apples and oranges. Eli Lilly and Co. could get away with the vague, unproven claim of greater safety because it's hard to make objective comparisons between drugs with different adverse effect profiles.

In Chapter 3 we saw that the stimulating effects of SSRIs are very common and extremely dangerous. In fact, Prozac has been shown to be a great danger in regard to one of the most serious adverse effects, mania. On this basis alone, it seems unreasonable to claim that SSRIs are safer than older antidepressants. But we haven't finished examining the harmful effects of the SSRIs. This chapter will discuss other adverse effects on the body. Then the following three chapters will look at SSRI-induced sexual and dysfunction, suicide, and violence.

Common Adverse Reactions in the Body[1]

In the Prozac label for 2001, a variety of adverse reactions are reported throughout the label without being compiled in any one place. This is part of the attempt to obscure the dangers of the drug. I have put together a table that combines information from various sources in the label (Table 4.1). As far as I can tell, no one has done this before, and therefore the overall data has been largely buried. The adverse effects listed in the table were considered "common" or "frequent" or they occurred in 2 percent or more of the patients and at a greater rate than among placebo patients. The percentage range in parentheses often reflects increased rates with rising doses. The table includes central nervous system adverse effects discussed earlier in the book.

Cardiovascular and Bleeding Problems

Beyond the common or frequent bodily adverse reactions listed in the table, the Prozac label lists a variety of others that are less frequent, including an array of cardiovascular disorders such as congestive failure, myocardial infarction, and potentially life-threatening arrhythmias. Some time ago, I noticed that there seemed to be an unusual number of heart-related reports being made to the FDA for SSRIs, in particular Zoloft, and I wrote to warn the FDA without receiving any response.

Recently Eli Lilly and Co. was about to release a new form of Prozac. Chemicals including drugs often come in right- and left-hand forms, mirror images of each other. The company wanted to market the right-handed mirror image as safer, but ended up withdrawing it from the approval process due to heart arrhythmias. There's been no apparent discussion of the implication for regular Prozac, approximately 50 percent of which is made from the right-handed form. Cardiac problems with the right-handed form demand a new look at the cardiac dangers of Prozac itself but the FDA hasn't shown any concern.

TABLE 4.1

Frequently Reported Adverse Effects of Prozac
Compiled from the 2001 Prozac Label

Nervous System		Digestive System	
Insomnia	16-33 %	Nausea	21-29 %
Anxiety	12-15 %	Diarrhea	12 %
Nervousness	11-14 %	Anorexia	8-17 %
Somnolence	13-17 %	Dry mouth	9-12 %
Dizziness	10 %	Dyspepsia	7-10 %
Tremors	10 %	Flatulence	3 %
Libido Decreased	3-11 %	Vomiting	3 %
Abnormal Dreams	1-5 %	Weight Loss	1.4-2 %
Agitation	frequent	Weight Gain	frequent
Amnesia	frequent	Increased Appetite	frequent
Confusion	frequent	Nausea	
Emotional Instability	frequent	and vomiting	frequent
Sleep Disorder	frequent		

Body as a Whole		Cardiovascular System	
Chills	frequent	Hemorrhage	frequent
Headache	21 %	Hypertension	frequent
Asthenia (Weakness)	9-21 %	Vasodilatation	3 %
Flu Syndrome	3-10 %	Palpitation	2 %
Fever	2 %		

Sensory System		Respiratory System	
Abnormal Vision	3 %	Pharyngitis	3-11 %
Ear Pain	frequent	Yawn	3-11 %
Taste Perversion	frequent	Sinusitis	1-6 %
Tinnitus	frequent		

Skin and Appendages		Urinary and Genital System	
		Impotence	2-7 %
Sweating	7-8 %	Abnormal Ejaculation	7 %
Rash	4 %	Libido Decreased	4 %
Pruritis (itching)	frequent	Urinary Frequency	frequent

Note: "Frequent" indicates at least 1 percent.

More Prozac Problems

The Prozac label also mentions several kinds of potentially fatal blood disorders, serious skin disorders, hypothyroidism, arthritis, leg cramps, acne, and hair loss. There is also a cluster of reports concerning abnormal menstrual cycles, menstrual bleeding, spontaneous abortion, and related problems. Prozac affects the serotonin in the platelets, small circulating bodies in the blood that control clotting, and there are many reports concerning abnormal bleeding on Prozac.

We have already noted the variety of gastrointestinal problems, including nausea, vomiting, stomach pain, anorexia, and weight loss. Especially after more lengthy exposure to SSRIs, unrelenting weight gain can become a serious problem.

Varying degrees of headache, muscular aches and pains, and feelings of weakness have been reported.

SSRIs cause rashes and increased sensitivity to sunlight. Sometimes rashes have been accompanied by dangerous systemic illnesses that include fever, elevated white blood cell count, joint pains and swelling, respiratory distress, and other signs of what looks like an autoimmune disorder. In a few cases, there has been serious involvement of the lung, kidney, or liver, leading to death. Prozac has caused fatal episodes that resemble anaphylactic shock with spasm of the bronchial tubes.

Animal studies with Paxil and Celexa have shown some potential for producing cancer. Several SSRIs have been shown to cause fetal and early developmental abnormalities or death in animals.

Hyponatremia (low blood sodium levels) has occurred on SSRIs possibly due to interference with ADH, a hormone that affects kidney function. During SSRI treatment the blood sugar may drop and after termination of treatment it may spike, complicating the treatment of diabetic patients.

Extrapyramidal Reactions and Tardive Dyskinesia

Extrapyramidal signs or symptoms, commonly called EPS, are abnormal movements caused by a variety of drugs. One common EPS is a Parkinsonian syndrome with flattened emotions and expression, tremor, rigidity, and impaired walking. Other EPS include muscle spasms (dystonias) and akathisia, the potential severe inner agitation that drives people to move about (Chapter 3). In an extreme manifestation of EPS, one that is often mistaken for a seizure, the patient's back and neck will spasm into a backward arc and the eyes may roll back in the head.

EPS are a well-known, extremely common adverse effect of neuroleptics or "antipsychotics," but EPS are also increasingly reported in association with taking the SSRI antidepressants.[2] SSRI drugs indirectly affect a neurotransmitter system called dopamine that plays a significant role in the development of EPS.

When an abnormal movement persists after the offending drug has been stopped, the disorder is called tardive dyskinesia—meaning "late-appearing movement disorder." The neuroleptics commonly cause a variety of permanent abnormal movements and spasms.

Tardive dyskinesia is one of the most devastating of all drug-induced disorders.[3] The abnormal movements or spasms can strike any of the muscles that are under voluntary control, including muscles of the face, eyes, mouth, tongue, neck, shoulders, arms, legs, hands, and feet. Breathing, speaking, and swallowing can also be impaired. One variant, called tardive dystonia, causes painful spasms, often in the neck and shoulders. Another, called tardive akathisia, involves excruciating agitation that compels the individual to move about. Both variants can produce lifelong physical and mental torture.

Tardive dyskinesia can vary from minimal to disabling, and is usually irreversible. In my clinical practice, I've evaluated cases of neuroleptic-induced tardive dyskinesia in which people were permanently disfigured, physically impaired, and exhausted by constant movement. There is no effective treatment.

In one malpractice case in which I was an expert, a woman's face and neck spasms were so painful and disfiguring, and the doctor's conduct so negligent, that the jury awarded her $6.7 million.[4] Her tardive dyskinesia resulted from being given a neuroleptic, Risperdal.

The rates for tardive dyskinesia are most thoroughly documented in regard to the older antipsychotic or neuroleptic drugs such as Thorazine, Navane, Mellaril, Prolixin, and Haldol. tardive dyskinesia will develop in 5 to 8 percent of neuroleptic patients for every year of exposure, so that after only three years, the risk of tardive dyskinesia is a monstrous 15 to 24 percent. For older people, the risk is even more astronomical and can exceed 20 percent per year.[5] Although the rates of tardive dyskinesia have not been as well established with the newer neuroleptics such as Zyprexa, Seroquel, and Risperdal, all of them pose the risk, and the FDA requires every one to make the same warning in its official label. Tardive dyskinesia is a tragedy of enormous proportions that has afflicted tens of millions of patients over several decades.

The risk of tardive dyskinesia from SSRIs remains controversial in part because drug companies have tried to minimize the problem. Among the SSRIs, Prozac has been available the longest and has been given to the greatest number of patients. As a result, Prozac has the most reports of tardive dyskinesia. Since tardive dyskinesia usually takes months or years before it becomes apparent, it is not surprising if it failed to show up in the short-term four-to-six-week trials. However, reports of abnormal movements during these trials should have alerted the drug company to the danger that some symptoms would become persistent in the form of tardive dyskinesia.

However, after marketing Prozac began, numerous Prozac-induced tardive dyskinesia reports caused the FDA to insist on some mention of the problem in the drug label. Under "Postintroduction Reports," the Prozac label now mentions the possibility of dyskinesia, but without confirming that the drug definitely causes it. Furthermore, the company avoids the dreaded term "tardive dyskinesia" and instead mentions only "dyskinesia." The Prozac label describes only one case in which the abnormal movements apparently cleared up.

Despite drug company attempts to minimize the problem, clinical reports of Prozac-induced tardive dyskinesia have been published[6] and many spontaneous reports have been sent to the FDA and Eli Lilly and Co. In fact, through September 30, 1991, Eli Lilly and Co. had already received thirty-five reports.[7] In my clinical practice, I have begun to see cases of SSSR-induced tardive dyskinesia.

Despite the frequency and potential severity of tardive dyskinesia caused by neuroleptics, the psychiatric and medical profession have taken decades to recognize its existence. Many doctors still refuse to take it seriously enough. Based on that history, tardive dyskinesia caused by SSRIs may turn out to be far more common and severe than originally estimated. However, the available evidence indicates that the rates for SSRI-induced tardive dyskinesia will be lower than for the neuroleptic drugs. Nonetheless, it poses a significant threat, and individual cases can be very traumatic to the victim.

Fertility, Pregnancy, and Nursing

All the SSRIs cross the placenta and therefore endanger the fetus, and are also found in the breast milk of nursing mothers where they threaten the infant.

Drug Facts and Comparisons reports that women taking Prozac in the first trimester have a significantly higher rate of birth defects (5.5 percent) and that women taking Prozac later in pregnancy more frequently give birth to premature infants (14 percent).[8] Some animal studies have shown decreased fertility on

SSRIs.[9] A study published in the *New England Journal of Medicine* found that infants exposed to Prozac in the third trimester had higher rates of premature delivery, more frequent admissions to special-care nurseries, and "poor neonatal adaptation, including respiratory difficulty, cyanosis [blue discoloring caused by lack of oxygenation] on feeding, and jitteriness."[10] The article continued, "Birth weight was also lower and birth length shorter in infants exposed to fluoxetine [Prozac] late in gestation."

Women who may become pregnant, who are pregnant, or who are nursing should never take these drugs. Remember that Prozac in particular has a long duration of action, and so it should be stopped five weeks or more before becoming pregnant.

SSRIs can interfere with having children in yet another way. As we'll see in the next chapter, these drugs can harm and even destroy love relationships and family life.

Pituitary Gland Dysfunction

A research team led by Margaret Johns (1982) from the Mount Sinai School of Medicine found serotonin-containing cells in the pituitary gland. The cells were located in the anterior or forward part of the gland where hormonal control takes place, including control of estrogen and testosterone.

Two years later, Johns and her colleagues (1984) demonstrated that Prozac *completely* blocks the uptake of serotonin by these pituitary cells.[11] In one examination, approximately 10 percent of pituitary cells were affected.

Johns's research goes a long way toward explaining how and why SSRIs cause so much sexual dysfunction. However, the implications of disrupting pituitary function are more extensive and more potentially disastrous. In response to the debate surrounding SSRI antidepressants, in July 2000 Johns wrote a letter to the editor of the *New York Times* that remains unpublished. She warned that the presence of serotonin in pituitary cells "suggests that serotonin normally plays a role in estrogen and testosterone production by regulating the release and/or synthesis of these pituitary hormones. These cells might not function well when deprived of serotonin. Their abnormal functioning could, in turn, have far reaching negative effects on blood vessels, bone, hair, and skin—and not just reproductive physiology and behavior—because all are influenced to some degree by estrogen and testosterone."

As in regard to most adverse effects of psychiatric drugs, experts in general, as well as the drug companies and the FDA, continue to pay remarkably little attention to these ominous findings.

Throughout the Body

Most people who take Prozac have not been told that serotonin, the substance that it interferes with, is spread throughout the body. Meanwhile, we have almost no understanding of the function of Prozac in the body. That's another reason to be wary of exposing yourself to SSRIs—functions throughout the body are being affected in ways we know little or nothing about.

Anyone who takes Prozac is causing largely mysterious biochemical changes throughout his or her body. In reality, we don't know much more about what serotonin does in the brain. It's worth reemphasizing that the serotonin chemical messenger network is so complex and so extensive, we would have to understand overall brain function to have any inkling about serotonin's specific role.

In the next chapter, we look at the devastating effects that SSRIs can have on sexual function and love life.

FIVE

How SSRI Antidepressants Can Ruin Love and Family Life

Mrs. Marcus asked her reluctant husband to come to therapy with her. He had been taking Prozac for several months and considered himself a kind of poster boy for the drug. He often told his friends and acquaintances how much it helped him and on one occasion had participated in a radio show with his psychiatrist to promote the drug.

As soon as he sat down in my office, it was obvious that Mr. Marcus was emotionally blunted and remote. He showed little expression and his voice lacked timbre.

"You look kind of flat to me," I said. "How do you feel?"

"I'm glad to be rid of feeling so bad," he answered.

We talked for a few minutes about what it meant to feel "so bad." It was hard for him to express himself but much of it surrounded conflicts with his wife and his previous wishes to get divorced.

"Does your psychiatrist notice that you've lost your spark?" I asked.

"I only see him for fifteen minutes every six weeks or so. I tell him I'm doing good and he writes me the prescription."

"He was never like this before," his wife burst out. "He used to be full of energy and vitality. He's only fifty, but he looks and acts like an old man. He seems *more* depressed to me. I even called his psychiatrist to tell him, and what did he do? He raised my husband's dose."

"I feel better than I used to," Mr. Marcus said without enthusiasm.

After a long pause, she blurted out, "We haven't made love in months!"

He shrugged and then said, "But we don't fight so much anymore. I couldn't stand the fighting. We were getting nowhere."

"We're not getting anywhere now," she explained sadly. "He knows this," she explained, "and I've been thinking of leaving. I can't stand to see him this way and it's making me feel like I'm not worth anything."

Mr. Marcus agreed to continue coming for therapy "for the sake of the marriage."

With his wife's encouragement over the next several weeks, he agreed to try gradually reducing his daily Prozac by one-third from 60 to 40 milligrams. Within a few weeks after the reduction, he began to brighten up. He asked for another reduction and then for an end to the medication. Within a few months, he felt like himself again for the first time since starting the medication.

Mr. Marcus found that even his memory function and his ability to think had been clouded on the drug without his perceiving it. In retrospect he saw that he not only lost his sex drive, he lost his interest in his wife and in almost everything and everyone else he cared about, when he was on the SSRI. He and his wife were making love again and arguing again, but now they were dealing with their conflicts in couples therapy and their life together was improving.

Impairing Our Self-Perception

Psychoactive drugs impair our ability to evaluate our own performance or experience, so it is easy for people to fool themselves about the benefits under their influence.

Remember the advertising campaign that urged us to stop drunken friends from driving by taking away their car keys? It's a good idea, of course, except that the inebriated friend is likely to resent us. People under the influence of alcohol tend to think they can drive as well as or even better than ever. Similarly, people who use alcohol or recreational drugs may believe at the time that they are improving their social and romantic life, but in reality they are relating in a superficial and sometimes foolish manner that's obvious to anyone who is not intoxicated.

After people stop taking recreational drugs or alcohol, they often realize in retrospect that the improvement in sex or in social relationships was illusory. The drugs or alcohol were covering up the superficiality or even the hostility and conflict in the relationships.

Although people taking SSRI antidepressants are not likely to believe or to claim that the drugs have improved their sex life, they are likely to minimize the devastating effects on their sexual function and on their love and family life. Their partners, like Mrs. Marcus, are more likely to tell the doctor about the problems created by the drug treatment.

Love and the Brain

Love requires a fully functioning brain. From alcohol and marijuana to psychiatric drugs, any psychoactive agent in the long run will dull awareness and disrupt intimacy. All psychiatric drugs can impair sensitivity, empathy, and caring, and as a result they can impair sexual experiences. As decribed in Chapter 4, SSRIs cause hormonal dysfunctions that directly impair the ability to experience or enjoy sex. In regard to impairing sex and love, SSRIs are in fact much worse than most psychoactive substances. Sexual dysfunction is a frequent SSRI effect.

The manifestations of SSRI-induced sexual dysfunctions are varied. Decreased desire or "libido" is very common in both males and females. Difficulties ejaculating are very frequent in men, as are difficulties reaching orgasm in women. Prolonged, painful erection of the penis, called priapism, has also been reported and is probably a rare event.

Based on their controlled clinical trials, Eli Lilly and Co. originally reported a sexual dysfunction rate of 1.9 percent for Prozac. In a separate part of a large chart, they listed decreased libido with a rate of 1.6 percent. As I pointed out in *Talking Back to Prozac*, splitting the data like this caused some doctors to underestimate the overall reported rate of 3.5 percent. But even 3.5 percent turned out to be a gross underestimate. Once again drug company–sponsored controlled clinical trials failed to demonstrate the true dangers associated with a drug. In subsequent published studies, reported rates for Prozac-induced sexual dysfunction in men range from 8 to 75 percent. The 75 percent figure came from one doctor's systematic queries of sixty consecutive patients.[1]

Probably because of the growing, inescapable awareness of the problem, more recent drug company clinical trials involving newer SSRIs have demonstrated higher rates of sexual dysfunction. The label for Paxil, for example, notes that 12.9 percent of men had problems ejaculating and another 10 percent had difficulties including impotence. In the Zoloft trials, 15.5 percent of men and 1.7 percent of women were reported to have sexual difficulties. Keep in mind that these are the rates for adverse reactions that were gathered and evaluated by the drug companies themselves, and that the real rates are undoubtedly higher.

Although reported rates vary widely, it remains apparent that SSRIs frequently disturb sexual function.

The Mechanism of SSRI Sexual Dysfunction

As documented in the previous chapter, serotonin can be found in the anterior pituitary gland that controls the synthesis and release of hormones such as testosterone and estrogen that play a central role in sexuality. Within the brain itself, serotonin nerves go to the thalamus and hypothalamus of the brain, where sexual regulation also occurs. Still other serotonin nerves end up in the frontal lobes, where they can influence the entire human experience of intimacy and love.

SSRIs indirectly disrupt dopamine nerves in the brain. Some researchers consider dopamine to be the "pleasure" chemical messenger. Although that's too simplistic, it draws attention to one route through which disruption of dopamine could impair sexual function.

Whatever the specific mechanisms, SSRIs make a large portion of people suffer from diminished feelings of love or sexual desire, and they cause impotence, delayed ejaculation, the inability to climax, and other sexual problems.

SSRI Indifference

Many people seem unconcerned about suffering from the sexual dysfunction that they experience when they take SSRIs. Partly that's related to the tendency of all psychoactive agents to impair judgment. It also results from a specific drug effect: SSRIs tend to cause a loss of interest in sex and in loving intimacy.

Adverse effects on sexuality tend to diminish at lower doses of the drugs and to go away entirely when the drugs are stopped. However, the damage done to the relationship may be lasting and even permanent.

I have treated men and women who threw away their marriages and other love relationships under the influence of SSRIs. Similarly, I have talked with spouses who reluctantly left their loved ones because of the effects these drugs were having on them.

A statistic on a table of adverse drug reactions cannot communicate the real toll in terms of damage to the quality of human life. Nowhere is this more apparent than in the arena of sexual dysfunction. Sexual dysfunction can cause a problem ultimately much larger and more important—love dysfunction. The combination of sexual and love dysfunction can and does ruin lives.

SIX

Depression and Suicide Caused by Antidepressants

Tally was a very bright, energetic woman who felt, if anything, that she had too much vitality. She was at times like a St. Bernard pup, trampling on people's feelings without realizing and barging into situations at work without thinking first. But her spontaneity and her lack of restraint endeared her to loved ones, including her boyfriend, and made her an excellent manager of people at work.

She had come to see me with her boyfriend to work out some difficulties before they got married. During the therapy, she went on vacation and suffered a skiing accident that resulted in considerable persistent physical pain in her back and neck. In an effort to control the pain, her orthopedic surgeon prescribed the SSRI Zoloft for her.

Tally had been on 100 milligrams of Zoloft for about six weeks when she decided it really wasn't helping her pain. If anything, she was beginning to feel depressed for the first time. She attributed her feeling "blue" to her pain and to her lack of exercise, and not to the Zoloft; but with little evidence that the Zoloft was helping, she decided to cut back on it.

The next day Tally's boyfriend called me and told me that she had reduced her Zoloft from 100 to 50 milligrams the day before, and that now, for the first time ever in her life, she was in a "black hole" and actively thinking of killing herself.

Tally and her boyfriend were in my office within hours. Nothing had happened in the last few days to make her feel so hopeless and despairing. The pain was no worse. She was able to carry on her life and even to sleep well at night with moderate amounts of painkillers. She couldn't give any explanation for why she wanted to die, but the feeling persisted.

Tally rejected the idea that she was "crashing" from the reduction in her medication. As someone who prided herself in taking charge of her own life and in being responsible, she argued that "a drug can't control my feelings." Nonetheless, she agreed to resume the 100-milligram dose of Zoloft and within an hour or two she felt like her normal self again. That convinced her she had been going through drug withdrawal.

Tally asked me to take over the prescription of her Zoloft and under careful supervision by me and her boyfriend, the drug was tapered and then stopped over a two-week period without any negative consequences.

Tally's story ended well in part because of my awareness of the tendency of SSRI antidepressants to cause suicidality, sometimes as a direct effect and, as in Tally's case, as a withdrawal reaction. Many other doctors, in my experience, would have increased her drug dose on the grounds she needed more of it. Or they would have added a second antidepressant that could have worsened her condition. I have been a medical consultant in many cases in which Prozac and other SSRI antidepressants have caused or contributed to suicide and to violence. If the FDA had been more responsible, these continuing tragedies could have been diminished in number or avoided. Psychiatrist Richard Kapit anticipated them when he was the chief medical officer at the FDA in charge of reviewing the dangers of Prozac prior to its approval.

The FDA Knew from the Beginning

When I began my review of FDA documents as a medical expert in product liability suits against Eli Lilly and Co., I was shocked and disillusioned by what I found. Until that time, I had not fully confronted the willingness of the FDA to protect drug companies, even at the cost of human life.

Behind the scenes at the FDA during the approval process for Prozac, Richard Kapit, the chief medical officer in charge of evaluating Prozac adverse effects, repeatedly warned that the drug might worsen depression in some patients. Chapter 3 described his concerns that "Prozac causes a set of adverse effects which resemble those caused by amphetamine,"[1] including agitation, insomnia, anorexia, and weight loss. In his lengthy "Safety Review" in March 1986, Dr. Kapit issued a serious warning: "Since depressed patients frequently suffer from insomnia, nervousness, anorexia, and weight loss, it is possible that fluoxetine [Prozac] treatment might, at least temporarily, make their illness worse." In his summary and conclusion, he reemphasized that "Depressed patients are often nervous, anxious, and sleepless, and they have often experience[d] loss of appetite and weight. It is possible, therefore, that fluoxetine may exacerbate certain depressive symptoms and signs." He added, "These problems should be examined in future studies of fluoxetine" and concluded his review with the suggestion that the label for the drug "advise physicians" about the danger of an "exacerbation" of depressive symptoms caused by Prozac.

The FDA systematically ignored these and many other warnings that Prozac could worsen depression. It did not require the company to mention any of these dangers in its label. Instead, as we shall see in this chapter, the FDA helped to expunge from the label the only indication of Prozac's tendency to worsen depression and the company in turn hid critical data from the FDA. Although the FDA did ask the company to conduct postapproval trials specifically aimed at evaluating the danger of Prozac-induced suicide, the company simply ignored the FDA, and nothing more was said about it by the government agency. From then on, Eli Lilly and Co. would act as if there were no basis whatsoever to be worried about Prozac worsening anyone's depression.

British, German, and French regulatory agencies were more responsible in dealing with their concerns about Prozac-induced stimulation leading to suicide.[2] The German and French agencies required some recognition of the problem in the official labels for the drug. In Great Britain, an editorial in the world's most prestigious medical journal, *Lancet*, warned that SSRIs were associated with "the promotion of suicidal thoughts and behavior," and more recently the British regulatory agency put a suicide warning on the label for Prozac.

In the United States, the FDA approved Prozac without requiring any warning from the drug company about stimulation and suicide. However, after Prozac was approved, hundreds of reports eventually led the FDA to require the company to mention the existence of "suicide" in association with taking Prozac without confirming that it was a proven adverse reaction.

Learning from Science and Clinical Experience

Like Tally, many people doubt that a medication can make a person suicidal or violent. It can be difficult to reconcile personal responsibility with the idea that a drug can make us act in a self-destructive or aggressive manner. When I first began to ponder these issues years ago, I believed that a drug could never make a person do anything that they didn't otherwise want to do. But as I learned more about the disruptive impact of psychoactive drugs on the mind, the issue grew more complicated, and after careful consideration I felt compelled by my scientific research and clinical experience to change my earlier conclusion. Under the influence of psychoactive chemicals, people can and do behave in ways that they would ordinarily reject as irrational or bad.

The final change in my understanding occurred when I was researching my medical book *Psychiatric Drugs: Hazards to the Brain* that was published in 1983. By the time I was finished with my background research, it was impossible to reject the idea that psychoactive drugs influence people to act in ways that their values and willpower would not normally allow. There were many sources of data to confirm these drug effects, including controlled clinical trials where people taking psychiatric drugs, compared to the same people taking a sugar pill, developed a variety of mental disturbances including depression, mania, and psychosis.

After the publication of my 1983 medical book, increasing numbers of patients began to consult me about their reactions to psychiatric drugs. My growing clinical and forensic experience confirmed that many kinds of drugs can produce extreme emotional responses, such as suicidal depression, violent agitation, and life-disrupting psychosis.

Many Drugs Cause Depression

Even drugs that are used in general medicine rather than psychiatry can cause dangerous degrees of depression. Recently I was consulted in the cases of men who committed suicide while taking the antiviral agent Rebetron for the treatment of hepatitis C. Initially the lawyer for the cases was skeptical about a drug causing or even contributing to suicidal feelings and actions. He was surprised when I read him the FDA-approved label for Rebetron in the *Physicians' Desk Reference* (2000). The following was bold and capitalized: "SEVERE PSYCHIATRIC ADVERSE EVENTS, INCLUDING DEPRESSION AND SUICIDAL BEHAVIOR (SUICIDAL IDEATION, SUICIDAL ATTEMPTS, AND SUICIDES) HAVE OCCURRED DURING [REBETRON TREATMENT] BOTH IN PATIENTS WITH AND WITHOUT PREVIOUS PSYCHIATRIC HISTORY."

Notice that these suicidal reactions were found in patients who had no prior psychiatric history, meaning they had no previous history of depression or suicidality.

Data from the clinical trials for Rebetron supported this warning. The research showed a 32 percent rate of depression after twenty-four weeks of Rebetron treatment, and an even higher 36 percent rate of depression at forty-eight weeks.

Although Rebetron is an extreme example, many drugs have been identified as causing depression. A review in 1990 *Health Letter* listed fourteen categories of drugs known to cause depression, including nonpsychiatric agents such as beta-blockers (Inderal), blood pressure drugs (Catapres, Aldomet, and Minipress), a variety of pain medications, and even some antibiotics.[3] The 1998 *Medical Letter* published a survey of "Some Drugs That Cause Psychiatric Symptoms." It listed more than 100 categories of medications and individual drugs that produced psychiatric reactions such as psychosis, hallucinations, confusion, delirium, depression, agitation, mania, and less commonly, suicidality and aggression.

Antidepressants, Mania, and Depression

As previously documented, many drugs including the SSRI antidepressants can cause mania. This has been proven in controlled clinical trials and in case reports, and is accepted in major textbooks and review articles. The American Psychiatric Association's *Diagnostic and Statistical Manual of Mental Disorders IV* (1994) is sometimes described as the "diagnostic bible" because of its widespread use for official purposes. As already noted the manual states unequivocally, "Symptoms like those seen in a Manic Episode may also be precipitated by antidepressant treatment such as medication . . . "[4]

In mania, as I've already described, the individual feels omnipotent, self-esteem is inflated, and blame is directed at other people for any problems the individual encounters. Aggressive behavior toward others is common. An otherwise law-abiding citizen may perpetrate criminal acts.

Depression is in many ways the opposite of mania. In depression, the individual feels helpless, self-esteem falls to a low ebb, and the individual blames himself or herself for any problems.

Aggression toward oneself is common. Instead of perpetrating criminal acts, the depressed person tends to feel guilty about relatively minor infractions.

Although mania and depression can be viewed as opposite sides of the same psychological coin, doctors are more willing to recognize drug-induced mania than drug-induced depression. Perhaps the production of mania seems more consistent with the idea that antidepressants help people by "elevating" their mood. They can view mania as a therapeutic effect that's become too exaggerated. But more important, drug-induced mania is such an obvious behavioral abnormality that it cannot be ignored when it surfaces for the first time during drug treatment. Therefore, it is more easily identified as an adverse drug reaction. Depression, on the other hand, is more subtle in its manifestations and easier to ignore or to blame on the patient's condition. But we'll find data confirming that antidepressants can cause an increase in both depression and in the suicide attempt rate.

Many drugs also cause psychotic symptoms. Stimulants, for example, have been known to make addicts psychotic and paranoid, sometimes in a dangerous fashion. The police get firsthand experience with how stimulant abuse leads to dangerously violent mental states. But even in prescribed doses used to treat children, stimulants can cause psychoses. A recent Canadian study reviewed a series of ninety-eight children diagnosed with ADHD who had been given Ritalin.[5] The retrospective analysis found a 9 percent rate of "psychotic symptoms" during Ritalin treatment. At the same clinic, no psychotic symptoms were reported in children with ADHD who did not receive Ritalin.

Prozac-Induced Suicide

Prozac was originally touted as safer than the older antidepressants because it is more difficult to commit suicide with a Prozac overdose. Although this is true, it does not take into account that Prozac and the other SSRIs increase the suicide rate, often producing particularly violent self-injury.

Prozac-induced acts of suicide are often especially brutal or bizarre, such as burning or stabbing oneself to death. I have found this in my forensic experience and it has been confirmed by a study of patients who committed suicide. According to a study done by Johns Hopkins and the Maryland coroner's office, patients who were taking Prozac tended to commit suicide in a more violent manner.[6] Taking SSRIs actually increases the likelihood of your intentionally harming yourself in a particularly violent and destructive fashion.

The danger of Prozac causing suicide became apparent to regulatory agencies in Europe. After Prozac was approved in the United States, the Germans remained reluctant to follow in our footsteps. The BGA, the German equivalent of the FDA, was receiving reports of increased suicide attempts in the European studies. The BGA asked Eli Lilly and Co. to review Prozac's earlier U.S.-controlled clinical trials to determine the rate of suicidal acts. The U.S. clinical trials compared Prozac to placebo and also to an older antidepressant, Elavil.

Eli Lilly and Co.'s own internal review found that the suicide attempt rate was indeed much higher for patients taking Prozac than for patients receiving the sugar pill or Elavil. In fact, suicide attempt rate was *six times higher* on Prozac than on placebo or Elavil. Even when taking into account that Prozac-treated patients were exposed to the drug for longer periods of time than the placebo- and Elavil-treated patients, Prozac patients attempted suicide three times more often.

Eli Lilly and Co. asked a sympathetic biopsychiatrist, David Winokur, to review their secret data. He wrote a memo explaining why Prozac might increase suicide. He observed, "Prozac might be somewhat more stimulating as a drug" and that the stimulation might be making the individuals "slightly more impulsive."

Although Prozac's manufacturer had been asked specifically to review this data for the German regulatory agency, the drug company never reported it to the Germans. When the company later defended itself before an FDA committee investigating Prozac and suicide, Eli Lilly and Co. continued to withhold the existence of its own damning study. I came upon the study while reviewing materials for discovery purposes as the medical and scientific expert in the initial series of law suits against the drug company.

More Evidence from Drug Company Data Confirming Antidepressant-Induced Suicide

Since my initial involvement in the product liability cases against Eli Lilly and Co., I've had the opportunity to examine the internal records of another company that makes an SSRI antidepressant. Once again the suicide rate appears to have been hidden, and the data indicates a higher rate of suicidality on the drug than on placebo.

Non-SSRI antidepressants can also increase the risk of suicide. After I briefed him on how to evaluate antidepressant suicide rates from drug company data, researcher Thomas Moore examined the suicide data for Serzone (nefazodone) and Effexor (venlafaxine) as generated during the FDA approval process.[7] Among 3,496 patients treated with Serzone there were 9 suicides and 12 suicide attempts, while among 875 placebo patients there were no suicides and only 1 suicide attempt. The suicide and suicide ratio was more than five times greater on Serzone than on placebo.

Moore made a similar analysis of Effexor. The suicide and suicide attempt ratio was almost three and a half times greater on Effexor than on placebo.

At first the reader may wonder, "But weren't the suicidal patients already feeling depressed?" However, the patient's depressed condition cannot account for the increased rate of suicide attempts on antidepressants such as Prozac, Serzone, and Effexor compared to placebo. All of the patients in the antidepressant trials were depressed, including those who were given placebo. Some of the studies even involved a crossover method in which the exact same patients were given the antidepressant and the placebo at different times. Both the antidepressant-treated and the placebo-treated patients were depressed, but the antidepressant-treated patients more often attempted suicide.

The "Smoking Gun"

As scary as these findings are, keep in mind that the drug companies control the entire reporting process and that the numbers of suicide attempts on the drugs are, in most cases, probably much larger than reported. In regard to Prozac-induced suicide, Eli Lilly and Co. systematically hid many reports that it received concerning suicide and suicide attempts. The drug company reclassified suicides as much more innocuous events, such as "no drug effect" or "depression." When a suicide was successful, the company would nonetheless label it as a "suicide attempt." When an attempt was later made to count the number of suicides on Prozac, the number counted would be much smaller than the actual number of suicides.

During the discovery process in which I participated for the initial Prozac suits, I came upon a most remarkable "smoking gun" indicating dissention and remorse among Eli Lilly and Co. employees concerning the fraudulent reclassification system. Claude Bouchy, a German employee of Eli Lilly and Co., protested the company's policy of reporting "suicide attempts" as "overdoses." Overdose is a term that can indicate accidental overdoses rather than active suicide attempts. Bouchy also protested reclassifying "suicidal ideation" into "depression" since contemplating suicide is more serious than feeling depressed. In a memo that went to a high-ranking U.S. official of Eli Lilly and Co., Bouchy protested, "I do not think I could explain to the BGA [the German FDA], to a judge, to a reporter or even to my family why we would do this especially on the sensitive issue of suicide and suicide ideation. At least not with the explanations that have been given to our staff so far."

Driving Patients to Suicide with Akathisia

All the SSRI antidepressants cause akathisia, that dreadfully distressing neurological stimulation and agitation discussed in Chapter 3.[8] Akathisia is key to many antidepressant-induced suicides. Akathisia feels even worse than ordinary anxiety and agitation. The experience is like being tortured from inside your own body by your own nervous system. I have seen akathisia drive people into feeling depressed, suicidal, and even violent. In discussing akathisia caused by other drugs, the American Psychiatric Association's *Diagnostic and Statistical Manual of Mental Disorders IV* (1994) makes the point that "Akathisia may be associated with dysphoria [painful emotions], irritability, aggression, or suicide attempts." It also mentions "worsening of psychotic symptoms or behavioral dyscontrol. . . . "[9] These are most remarkable admissions from the very heart of the psychiatric establishment.

Harvard Medical School psychiatrist Martin Teicher and his colleagues were among the first scholars to draw attention to the dangers of Prozac-induced akathisia in 1990 when they reported on a series of patients who became compulsively suicidal while taking the drug.

One year later, in 1991, Rothschild and Locke reported three cases of patients who made serious suicide attempts while taking Prozac and then recovered when the Prozac was stopped. To determine whether Prozac was the cause, the three patients resumed taking Prozac under close observation. They developed akathisia and explained that these distressing feelings had precipitated their original suicide attempts. The akathisia and the suicidal feelings abated once again when the Prozac was stopped for the second time.

In 1993 Teicher and his team published an extensive review of the literature confirming the relationship between Prozac and suicidal feelings. Then in 1994 I wrote further about the problem in *Talking Back to Prozac* (with Ginger Breggin) and presented additional data in 1997 in *Brain-Disabling Treatments in Psychiatry.*

There is now growing recognition of the danger of akathisia among informed doctors. For example, in 2000 psychiatrist Joseph Glenmullen wrote *Prozac Backlash,* a book that cites additional scientific literature updating what Teicher and I, and several others, initially observed.[10]

However, drug companies have done everything they can to obscure the problem and many doctors seem reluctant to take it into consideration or to warn their patients in advance. As a result, when patients then become agitated, upset, and potentially suicidal or even violent as a result of SSRI stimulation and akathisia, neither they nor their families have any idea that it could be drug induced. Their doctors may even increase the dosage of the drug, worsening the condition, and bringing about suicide attempts and violent acts.

Meanwhile, the FDA has allowed drug companies to systematically avoid collecting data on akathisia. A California court case in which I am an expert charges SmithKline Beecham with negligence by omission in failing to collect data on akathisia during its studies of Paxil for FDA approval.[11] Akathisia doesn't appear in Paxil's label until the paragraph entitled "Postmarketing reports," which contains adverse reactions reported to the company after the drug was put on the market.

Additional Reports Confirming Antidepressant-Induced Suicidality

David Healy is a psychiatrist in the United Kingdom who has followed up concerns originally expressed by me and by others about SSRI-induced suicidality. In a study published in 2000, Healy compared the effects of the SSRI Zoloft with those of another antidepressant, reboxetine, which has a different mechanism of action.[12] Each of twenty normal volunteers received one drug and then the other for two weeks each. They also had a drug-free interval in between. The study was double-blind; neither the volunteers nor the experimenters knew who was getting what drug.

Two of the previously normal subjects became depressed on reboxetine. More dramatically, on Zoloft two subjects developed "clear suicidal ideation, one of which reached extremely serious proportions." They both displayed a combination of akathisia and "emotional blunting." One of them came close to killing herself. She later reported that it seemed as if she could only "follow a thought . . . planted in her brain from some alien force." She was "jumpy, anxious and suspicious" and "her mind was racing and spiraling out of control." She described how "She suddenly decided she should go out and throw herself in front of a car, that this was the only answer." She was on her way out of the house when distracted from her trancelike state by a ringing phone. After stopping the Zoloft, she recovered after a few days.

A variety of other studies confirm that SSRIs increase the suicide rate. An epidemiological study in England showed increased rates of attempted suicide on Prozac compared with other antidepressants. A report from a county coroner in Texas showed an elevated rate of Prozac use among patients who killed themselves. In my own state of Maryland, as already noted, the coroner found that suicides involving Prozac were especially violent.[13]

Seeking a Suicide-Free Prozac

Lilly was planning to release a new form of Prozac by the beginning of 2002. The chemicals that make up drugs usually come in two mirror images called the right-handed and the left-handed forms. These forms can differ in their effects. The new form of Prozac would consist of the right-handed form, or R-fluoxetine.

The same Martin Teicher who authored the early report about Prozac-induced akathisia and compulsive suicidality became coinventor of the new form, along with Sepracor Inc., a Marl-borough drug company. Eli Lilly and Co. paid Sepracor Inc. for the rights to market the new drug.

Eli Lilly and Co.'s patent on Prozac was running out and com-petitors would be selling a lower-priced generic Prozac by August 2001. Although Prozac had global sales of $2.6 billion in 1999, it was down 7 percent from the previous year due in part to com-petition from newer SSRIs. The drug company needed a way to recapture the market with a brand-name drug similar to Prozac. The necessity for developing the new drug became critical to the survival of Eli Lilly and Co. in August 2000 when a judge ruled against extending the original Prozac patent, causing the drug giant's stock to plummet by 30 percent. Indeed, the impending threat of a generic Prozac caused a drop in the stock of other SSRI manufacturers as well.[14]

This "safer" variant was discarded in 2001 because it was found to cause abnormal heart rhythms, but not before Sepracor Inc. had begun a remarkable advanced marketing campaign in which it declared that the "new Prozac" would not produce sev-eral serious side effects of the "old Prozac," including "akathisia, suicidal thoughts, and self-mutilation."[15]

Making People More Depressed with Antidepressants

I was both surprised and shocked when I first stumbled on the fact that Prozac was making patients depressed. I found the data buried in the files at the FDA when I was looking at the final drafts of the label for Prozac. For many months before the drug was finally ap-proved, each revised draft of the Prozac label contained the obser-vation that the three most common adverse effects pertaining to the nervous system were "abnormal dreams, agitation, and depres-sion." This indicates that Eli Lilly and Co.'s clinical investigators frequently reported depression as an adverse effect of the drug.

If this information had remained on the label, it would have given some indication to health professionals that depressed patients might take a turn for the worse on Prozac. The label also mentioned agitation, and the combination of depression and agitation is known to be among the most dangerous mental states. It is frequently associated with suicidal and violent tendencies.

As I went through the cartons of material tracking the development of the label, I found a photocopy of the label as it was edited on the day that Prozac was finally approved for marketing. At the last minute, a high-ranking FDA official edited the entire label and drew a line through items he personally deemed unnecessary. Without explaining why he was deleting something as important as "depression" as a common adverse effect, he simply drew a line through it. There was no discernable scientific basis for this last-minute mutilation of data that had been developed over a period of many years.

No one reading the published label would know that drug company researchers found that depression was a common effect of Prozac. By a sleight of hand, "depression" as an adverse effect of Prozac went from "frequent" to nonexistent.

Meanwhile, the label for Paxil does list "depression" as one of the most frequently reported adverse effects on the brain and mind. However, the notation is somewhat lost in a list that reads: "Nervous System: *frequent.* Amnesia, CNS stimulation, concentration impaired, depression, emotional lability, vertigo." Also, the SSRIs had been on the market for a while at this point, and this sandwiched mention of "depression" as an adverse effect seemed to have no discernable effect on how doctors practice.

The Mechanism of Causing Depression and Suicide

Remember that Dr. Winokur, the consultant to Eli Lilly and Co., linked Prozac-induced suicide to the drug's stimulating effects. He suggested that the stimulation might make suicidal people more impulsive and hence more likely to act on their feelings. Indeed, it's been observed for decades that drugs that stimulate depressed people can drive them to suicide, and the SSRIs can have stimulating effects very similar to the effects of amphetamine, methamphetamine, and cocaine.

When people are depressed, they often want to die, but they usually lack the energy, drive, or motivation to do anything about it. If they get a burst of energy or stimulation, that can push them over the edge into acting on their impulses. Also, stimulation seems to loosen inhibition or self-control. People on stimulants can become emotionally unstable and unable to adequately control their emotions.

Even more important, when anxiety and agitation are added to feelings of depression the emotional state becomes especially intolerable and the desire to end one's life by suicide can grow. The mixture of depression and anxiety is called "agitated depression." As already mentioned, it's known to be associated with suicide and with violence.

Finally, as this book has amply demonstrated, the SSRIs commonly produce akathisia, that painful and even agonizing feeling of inner physical and emotional torment that can drive people to suicide or violence.

Antidepressants Do Not Prevent Suicide

Many doctors seem to believe that antidepressants will reduce the likelihood of a patient attempting or committing suicide. The labels for antidepressants warn about being careful about suicide but they emphasize that this care is required until the antidepressant can take effect. This falsely implies that antidepressants can reduce the danger of suicide.

After reviewing the vast literature and after examining the internal records of several antidepressant makers, it is absolutely clear that antidepressants do not reduce the suicide rate. It's a complete myth. If anything, as already demonstrated, taking antidepressants puts a person at greater risk for suicide.

SEVEN

Criminal Behavior and Violence Caused by Antidepressants

In both my clinical practice and in my medical legal work I have evaluated many cases of criminal activity and violence that seem unequivocally caused by psychiatric drugs. Although this may seem to many readers as a difficult case to prove, I believe this chapter will provide convincing evidence.

Playing at Being "The Saint"

Mr. Andrews was a man who was known among his friends and coworkers as an usually kind and gentle man.[1] It would be hard to find anyone who would make a criticism of him. His mother- and father-in-law felt as positively toward him as toward their own children. He had recently achieved a new and potentially very remunerative position selling insurance for a nationwide company through his own independent office.

Meanwhile, Mr. Andrews had gone to a doctor for help with his lifelong problem of obsessive worrying about whether he had offended someone's feelings. The doctor put him on Prozac and then shortly afterward added Xanax, a tranquilizer that, like Prozac, is known to cause mania and abnormal behavior.[2] In addition, Prozac raises the blood level of Xanax, greatly increasing its potentially toxic effects.

After several weeks, his family and friends began to notice a change in his behavior. He would watch video movies endlessly and he began to drink heavily for the first time in his life. SSRIs commonly lead people to increase their alcohol consumption, perhaps to control their stimulating effects.

Now he began to watch *The Saint,* a romanticized movie about a likeable thief. He became obsessed with these movies and even bought clothes to match the hero.

Then, with no previous history of criminal behavior or violence, he began a one-week series of several robberies that were bizarre and doomed to failure. First he robbed his wife's bank in their small community, driving his vintage blue Camero and wearing a mustache for a disguise. He was so cavalier about the robbery that he stood in front of the bank before the robbery discussing his car with a bypasser who, after the robbery, was able to describe the automobile down to its hubcap design.

Andrews escaped after the first robbery and returned home as if nothing had happened. He then went out and bought a trench coat, false beard, and sunglasses to go along with the character he was watching on his video.

For his last adventure, he robbed a bank near his mother's house. He was still driving his bright blue Camero. The police had been alerted to his activities a few minutes earlier when he entered a nearby Chinese restaurant without attempting to rob them nonetheless and frightened the staff with his outlandish false beard and outfit. While he ordered takeout food—which he forgot to take with him—they called the police.

Still wearing his disguise and carrying a pellet pistol with an empty CO_2 cartridge, he then robbed the bank. By the time the teller sounded the alarm, the police had already been alerted by the Chinese restaurant employees.

When Andrews came out of the bank, he ignored the police who were waiting for him with drawn guns. He robotically marched by them, got into his vintage blue car, and drove off in a hail of bullets. A short time later, he surrendered without a fight.

Later in the day when he was in jail he told his wife that he was worried. Why was he worried? He was afraid he'd miss a business appointment the following day.

After being taken off Prozac and Xanax, Andrews quickly returned to normal. He was at a complete loss in regard to explaining his strange behavior. Except for the disastrous consequences of his actions, he would have been able to continue his life as if nothing had happened.

I wrote a report for the defense stating that Andrews was suffering from a Xanax- and Prozac-induced manic episode that caused his criminal and violent behavior. A Harvard psychiatrist hired by the prosecution confirmed that Prozac caused his criminal behavior. The prosecution conceded and the court found him not guilty by reason of insanity caused by psychiatric drugs, especially Prozac.

After he was released from jail, Andrews continued to seek psychiatric treatment and to work. His family life continued to prosper.

Two years later, it was time for Andrews's sentencing hearing. Although he had been acquitted of any crime on the grounds of drug-induced psychosis, he was required to submit himself to a thirty-day evaluation in the state facility for the criminally insane. He was ripped out of his work and family life and put into a state psychiatric facility for the criminally insane.

Unfortunately, political circumstances had changed. Eli Lilly and Co. had now learned about the case. The company went to the prosecution to offer help in doing everything they could to salvage Prozac's reputation. Among other things, the drug company helped guide the prosecution in how to conduct their part of the sentencing hearing. The drug company also embarrassed the judge by ridiculing his decision in the local press. Meanwhile, the state psychiatrists now claimed that—despite the opinions of the original experts and the judge—Andrews would not have become manic unless he had manic tendencies. They had no scientific or medical basis for this claim (Chapter 3). Prozac can make people manic without a past history of mania.

Despite having caused no problems whatsoever during the two years between his release and his sentencing, the judge sentenced him to a potentially lengthy sentence in the facility for the criminally insane. He could be there for ten years.

Rarely have I been so saddened by the outcome of a hearing or a trial. Rarely have I been so outraged by the conduct of a corporation as by Eli Lilly and Co.'s determination to sacrifice this decent man to their own interests.

Eli Lilly and Company tell reporters that the "Prozac defense" has never worked. The case of Andrews shows that, to the contrary, a judge has clearly endorsed this defense by finding him not guilty as a result of intoxication with Prozac. During the sentencing hearing, the judge also made clear that he had considered Prozac, rather than Xanax, to be the main culprit. That Andrews ended up with a long incarceration for "treatment" is strictly the result of Eli Lilly and Co.'s effect on the prosecution and the judge during the sentencing phase.

In addition to Andrews's case, I have been involved as a medical expert in other cases in which a jury and prosecuting attorneys have been influenced by the "Prozac defense" to give lesser sentences for crimes committed under the influence of Prozac.[3]

Taking Care of the Dog

In a surprisingly similar case, I testified during a sentencing appeal and once again the judge accepted my viewpoint that the medication had caused or contributed to the criminal activities. Like Andrews, Mr. Blane committed bizarre robberies under the influence of Paxil as well as tranquilizers, and like Andrews, he had no criminal record.

Blane was a financial consultant earning almost six figures, but he was experiencing severe family stress. He was prescribed the antidepressant Paxil and the tranquilizer Restoril (temazepam) as a sleeping medication.

Blane was in the habit of taking his lunch break by driving into a pleasant area of the surrounding community, parking his car, and eating a sandwich. On one occasion, he saw a dog playing in a nearby yard. He went into the yard and petted the dog. The dog seemed hungry and, with no awareness of acting dangerously or bizarrely, Blane opened the unlocked back door of the house with the intention of finding a snack for the dog. Once inside, he took a doggie snack from the refrigerator and then sat down at the kitchen table to look over his office work while he finished his lunch. Before leaving, he went to the bathroom, happened to find a bottle of prescription pain medication, and stole it. He took nothing else.

For several days in a row, Blane repeated this pattern. He would walk into houses to eat his lunch, do a little office work at the kitchen table, and steal any pain pills that were in the bathroom cabinet. He took nothing else from the homes. He wore no gloves, left fingerprints everywhere, and on the last occasion, left some of his papers behind.

During one of these intrusions, a neighbor heard him break the back door windowpane, and—since he was parked in front of the house—was easily able to get Blane's automobile license number. Blane repeated his lunchtime forays in the same neighborhood over a few days, so that the police were able to lay in wait for him. He was caught with the prescription bottles in open view in the backseat of his car with the names of owners on them.

Was Blane a stupid man? No, he's actually one of the most intelligent people I know—a whiz in the financial arena. He is also a very good man. Would he have behaved this way "in his right mind"? Of course not. He was in a maniclike psychotic state caused by the psychiatric drugs.

By the time I entered the case, Mr. Blane had remorsefully confessed and was serving a lengthy jail sentence. My report during a sentence reevaluation hearing convinced the judge that Blane had been under the influence of Paxil at the time of the crimes. The judge shortened Blane's sentence and released him into private treatment.

I could devote a book to cases of drug-induced bizarre behavior. Often the crimes are relatively minor but nonetheless disastrous in terms of the individual's self-worth, reputation, and future. A respected corporate executive shoplifted for the only time in his life when he was taking Prozac. Directly in front of a store surveillance camera, he switched the price labels on a pair of baseball shoes and a bat. The prices were obviously inconsistent with the items, and he was easily caught as he checked out. After he was apprehended, it took him several minutes to realize he had done something seriously wrong. A man with a high income and a good future pension, he hardly needed to save a few dollars in this manner. He felt confused and humiliated by what he had done. His professional future was severely threatened.

Ending in Physical Violence

In the stories I have recounted, no physical harm was perpetrated. However, in my clinical practice and my medical legal work, I have evaluated many cases of drug-induced violent behavior. George was an especially tragic case. He, too, was a man with no history of violence who loved his wife and children. When he became depressed, his doctor put him on Paxil. Within three days, he had drowned his two young children and himself in their bathtub.

The family has brought charges of negligence against the drug company, SmithKline and Beecham, for allegedly failing to warn that Paxil can have serious adverse effects after the first dose, and that it can cause suicide and violence. I'm an expert in this ongoing case.

Children can also be driven to violence by SSRIs. A shy, rather meek fourteen-year-old girl who had never handled a gun found a long-forgotten family pistol and fired it pointblank at a boy who had been harassing her. Fortunately, it did not go off. She had been depressed and taking Prozac. My testimony led the jury to convict her of a lesser crime than the state demanded.

A man who was described as a Boy Scout by friends was given Prozac when he became distressed during a separation from his wife. He became extremely agitated on the Prozac, burst into his estranged wife's home carrying a pistol, and dragged her out of the shower. He then realized he was behaving insanely and stopped what he was doing. It was the only act of violence in his entire life. My report led the prosecution to reach a plea bargain in which the man did not have to spend any time in jail.

A man with severe back pain became addicted to analgesics and then was treated with a hodgepodge of psychiatric drugs, including antidepressants. In a fit of rage, he brutally assaulted his wife with a knife and killed her. In several cases of bizarre out-of-character incidents of violence like this, I have found this particular pattern of back pain and disability leading to the prescription of multiple painkillers and psychiatric drugs. In this case, the jury again convicted him of a lesser crime than the state requested.

In another case, Vance was prescribed Remeron, a relatively new antidepressant that affects several neurotransmitter systems. He was feeling agitated and depressed over marital conflicts, and after beginning the Remeron, his condition worsened. He began to have maniclike racing thoughts, paranoid feelings, and violent impulses. He assaulted his wife in an extremely brutal manner in front of multiple witnesses.

Vance was convicted of murder without his defense attorney bringing up the adverse effects of Remeron as a defense or even as a mitigating circumstance. Attorneys in criminal cases often have no idea that psychiatric drugs can contribute to abnormal, irrational, bizarre, and destructive behavior. I have written a report on his behalf and we are awaiting the response of the court.

In many cases of violent assault, prosecuting attorneys, judges, and juries are reluctant or unwilling to accept the idea that drugs can cause or worsen an individual's behavior. As a result, in some cases my testimony has not resulted in a reduction in the verdict or the charges. Also, Eli Lilly and Co., the manufacturer of Prozac, puts the full force of its influence into any courtroom in which a defendant raises a "Prozac defense." The defendant not only ends up having to contend with the resources of the state prosecutors but with the resources of the multibillion-dollar company that provides research and even a courtroom script for how to defeat the Prozac defense. I'll talk more about this in my chapter on the politics of antidepressants, including my participation in a famous trial surrounding the case of Joseph Wesbecker, who committed mass murder at his former place of work under the influence of Prozac. In that case, as we shall see, Eli Lilly and Co. was caught fixing the trial.

A Natural Desire to Hold People Responsible

There is a natural desire to hold people responsible for criminal or violent behavior. I share this desire to emphasize human responsibility. But as I've documented in the earlier chapters, antidepressants are known to cause psychosis and mania. That alone confirms that psychoactive drugs can severely impair mental function. When the brain is disrupted, and especially when it is overstimulated, people can lose their ability to control their behavior or to make accurate judgments about what they are doing. At the least, they are not as mentally equipped to make decisions as they would be with intact brains that were not suffering from psychosis or other disorders.

These drug-induced reactions are not "mental disorders" or "mental illnesses" in the vague way that those terms are bandied about. Drug-induced manic reactions or psychoses are genuine physical disorders. They are better described as neurological diseases or impairments than as mental disorders. In earlier years, they were called "organic psychoses" to distinguish them from "nonorganic" problems such as schizophrenia or manic-depressive disorder. But nowadays organized psychiatry has purposely blurred the distinction between known physical disorders, such as Alzheimer's or a drug-induced psychosis, and problems such as schizophrenia or depression with no known physical cause.

Drug-induced psychoses are directly rooted in drug-induced brain dysfunction. They are genuine brain disorders like Alzheimer's or Parkinsonism rather than "mental illnesses" like depression or panic disorder.

Antidepressants, Mania, and Violence

It should now be apparent from earlier chapters that all antidepressants, including the SSRIs, can cause mania. As previously documented, Prozac can cause mania in patients with no prior tendency toward mania. It is worth quoting once again from the American Psychiatric Association's *Diagnostic and Statistical Manual of Mental Disorders, IV* (1994), when it observes, "Symptoms like those seen in a Manic Episode may also be precipitated by antidepressant treatment such as medication."[4]

The diagnostic manual also makes clear that mania is commonly associated with violence and other criminal acts, and that the behavior, although psychotic, can be very purposeful or "goal-directed." For example, the diagnostic manual states patients often display "irritability, particularly when the person's wishes are thwarted." Furthermore, the individual may experience "negative consequences of actions that result from poor judgment (e.g., financial losses, illegal activities, loss of employment, assaultive behavior.)" Note especially the mention of "illegal activities" and "assaultive behavior." The description of mania also notes that "Some individuals, especially those with psychotic features, may become physically assaultive or suicidal." The manual also notes, "Mood may shift rapidly to anger or depression." These statements occur in the same section entitled "Manic Episode" in which it is stated that antidepressants can cause mania.

As described earlier, the American Psychiatric Association's *Diagnostic and Statistical Manual of Mental Disorders* is the official source for diagnosis in psychiatry. It is used in most research, in the FDA approval process, and by insurance carriers. Furthermore, the material in the manual reflects a consensus among recognized experts in the particular area that is being discussed. Given that this conservative diagnostic manual makes clear that antidepressants cause mania and that mania can produce goal-directed criminal acts, anger, violence, depression, and suicide, no physician should doubt that antidepressants cause acts of violence or suicide. Unfortunately, despite clinical experience, scientific data, and a consensus of opinion among experts, many doctors refuse to believe that their medications are sometimes driving patients to crime, violence, and suicide.

The Danger of Agitated Depression

A person suffering from agitated depression—a combination of depression and anxiety or irritability—is especially prone to aggression or violence. The individual is both depressed and stimulated, a very distressing state of mind, and one with sufficient energy to take action. In most cases of antidepressant-induced violence that I have examined, the individual was suffering from an agitated depression before the drug treatment was started. Often the antidepressant obviously worsened the agitated depression, resulting in suicide, murder, or both.

As the stories in these chapters confirm, drug-induced violence can occur at almost any time, including the first few doses of an

SSRI. In my experience, they most commonly occur when the drug is being started, increased, or stopped—that is, during changing levels of the drug in the blood stream.

FDA Recognition of
Drug-Induced Violence

A number of FDA-approved antidepressant labels acknowledge reports of hostility, aggression, or violence, as well as mania and paranoia that can contribute to violence. Without acknowledging a definite causal connection, the label for Prozac, for example, mentions many severe abnormal mental reactions that have been reported in association with taking Prozac, including psychosis, antisocial reaction, delusions, hallucinations, suicide, and violence. As another example, the Paxil label mentions central nervous system stimulation, depression, and emotional lability as occurring frequently. It then lists abnormal thinking, delirium, euphoria, manic reaction, paranoid reaction, and hostility as occurring infrequently.

I already described how Remeron, an atypical antidepressant, probably worsened one individual's depression and agitation and probably caused or contributed to his violence. The Remeron label summarizes adverse reaction reports from the total database of patients treated in clinical studies. Under the category of nervous system, depression, agitation, and anxiety are listed as frequent, whereas depersonalization, delirium, delusions, hallucination, manic reaction, emotional lability, euphoria, paranoid reaction, and hostility are listed as infrequent.

The warnings section on the Remeron label states that the incidence of mania during drug treatment was 3 in 1,000. Although this might seem relatively low to the layperson, mania is extremely dangerous, causing the FDA to require its inclusion in a special warning section. Also, as previously emphasized the rates for mania will be much higher in actual clinical practice where the patients are more varied, drug combinations are more dangerous, and monitoring is much less careful.

Wellbutrin (buproprion), yet another so-called atypical antidepressant that affects several neurotransmitters, can have very stimulating effects. It commonly drives the brain to the point of precipitating seizures. As its official label indicates, even in the short-term controlled clinical trials Wellbutrin caused increased rates for agitation (31.9 percent), insomnia (18.6 percent), anxiety (3.1 percent), and hostility (5.6 percent). In its larger database, mania/hypomania, depression, and hallucinations were "frequent" in individuals taking Wellbutrin. Paranoia was infrequent.

The precautions section for Wellbutrin is unusually strong in warning about stimulating effects, including agitation and insomnia. It states, "A substantial proportion of patients treated with WELLBUTRIN experience some degree of increased restlessness, agitation, anxiety, and insomnia, especially shortly after initiation of treatment." The precautions section also warns in bold print about the Wellbutrin-induced "Psychosis, Confusion, and Other Neuropsychiatric Phenomena," specifically including paranoia. The section also warns about the danger of "Activation of Psychosis and/or Mania." This stimulant syndrome is a prescription for aggression and violence.

Drug Mechanisms for Causing Violence

Many of the most obvious cases of drug-induced violence involve mania. However, mania is by no means the only way antidepressants can induce violence.

The SSRI antidepressants, as well as some other antidepressants such as Wellbutrin and Desyrel (trazodone) cause akathisia. In earlier chapters, I described this drug-induced neurological condition that can become a virtual inner torture of irritation and anguish. Akathisia can drive a person toward bizarre and even violent actions. SSRIs can also cause a loosening of inhibition or self-control, leading to unanticipated acts of violence.

Epidemiological Evidence from the FDA

Because drug-induced violence is relatively uncommon, it's difficult to study large enough populations to demonstrate a connection between any drug and violence. However, the FDA carried out an epidemiological study based on voluntary reports sent to it after Prozac was put on the market. The FDA reviewed all of the reports it had received concerning Prozac-induced "hostility" and "intentional injury" and presented the data at a 1991 FDA hearing on the subject of antidepressant-induced suicide. Although of critical importance, the data was merely mentioned in passing as part of a slide presentation and was then completely ignored. When I sought the data through freedom of information, the FDA claimed to have lost it.

However, I received a second opportunity as a medical expert to obtain the data from Eli Lilly and Co. under court order. I then testified about it in the Wesbecker murder-suicide case.[5] The FDA study compared the number of reports of "hostility" and "intentional injury" for Prozac to the number of reports for another antidepressant, trazodone. Even taking account of the greater number of prescriptions for Prozac, reports for hostility and intentional injury were eight times higher for Prozac than for trazodone. Furthermore, this avalanche of reports related to aggression and violence began to pour into the FDA before the controversy became public. Therefore, it was not the result of the publicity that was later generated around the subject of Prozac and violence. The reports were genuinely spontaneous, mostly from doctors and hospital pharmacists.

Clinical experience confirms that most antidepressants commonly cause a stimulant syndrome and akathisia, and that these can cause or exacerbate violent behavior. Many patients actually become manic, psychotic, and paranoid on antidepressants, and these mental conditions can result in various kinds of criminal activities, including bizarre robberies and aggression and violence. These antidepressant-induced abnormal behaviors are often out of character, unexpected, highly irrational, and sometimes brutal. Antidepressant studies carried out for FDA approval often generate data that confirm the production of the stimulant syndrome, akathisia, psychosis, mania, and paranoia. Hostility and violence are also mentioned in the FDA-approved labels for some antidepressant drugs.

The antidepressants as a group have a dangerous potential to produce abnormal behavior that can culminate in both suicide and violence. The SSRI antidepressants are especially liable to produce extremely irrational and sometimes horrendously violent acts.

EIGHT

Dangerous Drug Interactions and a Genetic Vulnerability to Severe SSRI Toxicity

There are so many potential hazards involved in taking SSRIs that no physician is capable of remembering all of them and no patient can be adequately informed about the dangers without spending days or weeks reviewing the subject in a medical library. Even this book cannot provide a thorough summary of all the problems. However, this chapter will discuss some of the more serious and exotic dangers associated with taking SSRIs.

The Serotonin Syndrome: Much Too Much of a Supposedly Good Thing

The serotonin syndrome resembles an extreme form of SSRI overstimulation, including irrational euphoria (maniclike symptoms), agitation, confusion, and gastrointestinal problems, such as diarrhea. However, it also involves whole body and neurological symptoms, such as fever and chills, poor coordination, muscle spasms, and hyperactive reflexes. It can manifest in a variety of confusing ways, can vary from mild to severe, and sometimes results in death.

Any SSRI can cause a serotonin syndrome, but it more commonly occurs when SSRIs are combined with other drugs that also stimulate serotonin. The antidepressants called MAOIs[1]— Parnate (tranylcypromine), Nardil (phenelzine), Marplan (isocarboxazid), and Eldepryl (selegiline)—can become lethal when mistakenly combined with SSRIs. MAOIs should be stopped at least two weeks before starting an SSRI, and MAOIs should not be started until at least five weeks after discontinuing an SSRI.

Many other drugs can interact with SSRIs to cause the serotonin syndrome, including tryptophan; psychostimulants such as the amphetamines and Ritalin; buspirone (BuSpar); lithium; and amantadine and bromocriptine. A variety of older antidepressants that stimulate serotonin can also cause a serotonin syndrome. I have been a medical consultant in cases in which combining SSRIs with a drug such as Elavil (amitriptyline) has resulted in death.

More than the Liver Can Handle

Most drugs, including the SSRIs, are broken down or metabolized by the liver before they are excreted from the body by the kidneys. The liver contains an enzyme system called P450 with many subtypes that participate in the metabolism of drugs.

Some drugs, including the SSRIs, tend to inhibit the activity of one or more of these P450 enzymes. This inhibition can prevent the rapid metabolism and elimination of any drug taken at the same time that depends on the enzyme for its degradation. This can lead to an extreme increase in the blood level and hence toxicity of the second drug.

Prozac, for example, can raise the blood concentrations of several types of drugs to dangerously high levels, including antidepressants such as Elavil (amitriptyline); benzodiazepine tranquilizers such as Xanax; Tegretol (carbamazepine); and antipsychotics such as Haldol and Clozaril.

Paxil is particularly potent in inhibiting a P450 enzyme and therefore increases the risk involved in taking a variety of medications that depend on the enzyme for their degradation in the body.

All of the SSRIs can inhibit one or another liver enzyme, and overall there are far too many potentially dangerous drug interactions to review in this book. Indeed, there are too many harmful drug interactions for any practitioner to keep track of. This is one more reason to avoid prescribing or taking these drugs. However, any doctor who prescribes SSRIs and any patient who receives them should take the time to review potentially dangerous drug interactions listed in books such as the annual *Drug Facts and Comparisons*.

A Missing Enzyme in the Liver

In the previous section, I described how liver enzymes are required to metabolize or break down SSRIs. Unfortunately, some people have a genetic makeup that lacks one or another of the key enzymes involved in metabolizing or breaking down specific SSRIs. Therefore, the drug will stay in their bodies in higher concentrations for longer periods of time. Because blood levels are increased, the risk of toxicity of almost any kind, including psychosis or a serotonin syndrome, is increased.

This potentially lethal vulnerability to overreacting to SSRIs is surprisingly common. An estimated 7–10 percent of Caucasians lack the major enzyme in the liver responsible for breaking down or destroying the SSRIs and some of the other antidepressants as well. The enzyme is also missing in approximately 3 percent of African Americans and 1 percent of Arabs and Asians.[2]

The missing enzyme is called P450 CYP2D and it plays the key role in breaking down many kinds of medications. People who lack the enzyme are called "poor metabolizers" because their body does not adequately destroy the drug. Indeed, people missing this enzyme have only one-ninth the ability of other people to degrade these drugs and eliminate them from the body. As a result, a routine dose of Prozac or almost any antidepressant can cause a very severe and even potentially fatal reaction.

Recently, a nine-year-old boy died of seizures and cardiac arrest after taking several psychiatric drugs at high doses, including Prozac.[3] On autopsy, the level of Prozac in the body was so extremely high that the parents were accused of poisoning him. However, further analysis revealed that the child was one of the 7–10 percent of white people who lack the gene that makes the enzyme.

This warning cannot be made too emphatic: A significant percentage of the population is genetically vulnerable to severe toxic reactions to antidepressants such as Prozac and other psychiatric drugs—but potential patients are rarely informed about this possibility before they take these drugs.

Doctors themselves often lack an appreciation of the seriousness of the problem. The official label for Prozac mentions that "a subset (about 7%) of the population" has a "reduced" activity of this enzyme, but the text is too difficult to understand and plays down the problem. If this problem were taken with sufficient seriousness, no one would take such psychiatric drugs without first being tested for the liver enzyme and, in fact, for a number of other enzymes that also affect drug metabolism. Instead, so little attention has been given to the problem that it is almost impossible for a physician to find a laboratory that will test to see if the enzyme is missing before prescribing SSRIs. Although I am in contact with a research laboratory that can perform the test, I have been unable to locate a commercial laboratory that will do them routinely for physicians.

More than the Plasma Proteins Can Contain

Not all drugs circulate freely in the blood stream. Many are bound to proteins in the blood. When a drug is bound to plasma proteins, it remains temporarily unavailable and therefore inactive. SSRIs have a tendency to bind especially tightly to circulating proteins, leaving less binding room for other drugs. As a result, other drugs will circulate more freely in the blood and have a greater than expected effect. The list of potential interactions is so extensive that most textbooks don't even try to list them all. They have to be checked on a drug-by-drug basis in sources such as the annual *Physicians' Desk Reference,* but this is a tedious process and the results are not necessarily comprehensive.

Overall, I hope that physicians and patients alike who read this book will approach SSRI antidepressants with much greater caution than is now customary among professionals and consumers.

NINE

Special Dangers of
Treating Children with SSRIs

"My son has been diagnosed as bipolar. They want to give him even more psychiatric drugs." In the last few years, I have heard this anguished communication innumerable times in clinical evaluations, conferences, on radio talk shows, on the telephone, and on my e-mail.

Bipolar disorder is the new name for manic-depressive disorder. For the first time in the 100-year span that the diagnosis has existed, it is being freely applied to children.

In almost every case that I have evaluated, the child displayed no symptoms of "mania" until being placed on a stimulating drug such as Ritalin and Adderall or an SSRI antidepressant. Every stimulant and every antidepressant can cause mania, and they are especially prone to do so in children. These children do not have "bipolar disorder," they are suffering from drug-induced mania. There is almost never reason to believe that they would have developed mania without being driven into it by a stimulating drug.

Tragically, instead of being taken off the offending drug, thousands of children are being given additional drugs to control the "mania." This often worsens their condition by making them apathetic and depressed. By the time I see these children, they may be taking four or five drugs, all of them absolutely unnecessary. In a theme that bears repeating throughout this book, the children improve as they are removed from their drugs. They become more able to listen and learn from their parents and more able to control their behavior. Their parents in turn can more quickly observe the improvements in their child's life that quickly follows improvements in their parenting techniques and in the child's school situation.

Growing Numbers of Children on SSRIs

There's no national databank on how many children and teenagers are being prescribed SSRIs and other antidepressants, but the number is almost certainly in the hundreds of thousands and growing. A study published in the *Journal of the American Medical Association* showed an increase in giving these drugs to two- to four-year-old toddlers.[1]

Meanwhile, no drugs are FDA-approved for depression in children. Luvox is approved for obsessions and compulsions in children but not for depression. Other than that, the FDA has not given its imprimatur to any use of SSRIs for any purpose in children.

There are two reasons why SSRI antidepressants are not FDA-approved for children: They don't work and they are very dangerous. As a result of my product liability work, I am able to look into the files of drug companies, and I can affirm that some of them tried to get their drug approved for children but were unable to do so.

Hazards to the Child's Brain

When it was revealed in the *Journal of the American Medical Association* that SSRIs are being given in increasing numbers to children, editor and psychiatrist Joseph Coyle (1997) raised serious concerns about giving these drugs to children. He showed special concern about exposing the growing brains of children to agents that distort the biochemical reactions that control the way the brain will develop.

Until recently there were few if any actual studies of how these drugs impact the growing brain. Now studies have begun to confirm the obvious—that SSRIs are not good for growing young brains. As reviewed in Chapter 2, a 1999 project gave Prozac to very young rats for two weeks.[2] The exposure to Prozac resulted in lasting and probably permanent brain abnormalities in serotonin nerves in the frontal cortex—the area of highest evolutionary development in the mammalian brain and the seat of intelligence, judgment, love, and all other higher functions.

An MRI brain scan study of children showed shrinkage in the brains of children who were taking the SSRI antidepressant Paxil for the treatment of obsessive-compulsive disorder.[3] The authors of the study waffled about cause and effect, but their data should be seen as a large red flag warning about a high probability of permanent brain damage from SSRIs. The young brain seems especially unable to handle the biochemical imbalances created by these drugs.

The Vulnerability of Children to Adverse Reactions

The SSRIs commonly cause serious adverse reactions in children with especially disastrous impacts on their mental life and behavior. Scientific reports are so convincing that no informed doctor should give these drugs to a child. In 1990–1991, for example, a group of Yale doctors found that 50 percent of children from ages eight to sixteen developed two or more abnormal behavioral reactions to Prozac.[4] Drug-induced reactions included aggression, loss of impulse control, agitation, and maniclike symptoms. The effects lasted until the Prozac was stopped.

Doctors from the University of Pittsburgh took a retrospective look at clinic charts of youngsters from age eight to nineteen who had taken Prozac.[5] They found that an extraordinary 23 percent of Prozac-treated young people developed mania or "maniclike" symptoms. Remember, mania is an extremely destructive reaction, potentially involving life-threatening, irrational behavior that can ruin a child's life. Another 19 percent of this group of children developed drug-induced hostility and aggression, including a "grinding anger with short temper and increasing oppositionalism." These are very discouraging results.

A controlled clinical trial conducted at the University of Texas found that Prozac caused a 6 percent rate of mania in depressed children ages seven to seventeen. The reactions were severe enough to require the children to drop out of the trials.[6] By contrast, none of the depressed children who took placebo (sugar pill) developed mania. Therefore, the mania was caused by the Prozac rather than by the mental condition of the children.

Confusing the Issue of
Drug-Induced Mania in Children

Doctors who prescribe psychiatric drugs to children often attribute their drug-induced mania or depression to some previously hidden defect in the children themselves. They frequently speak of the drug causing the mania to "emerge" as if it would have happened anyway in the future. That is, instead of recognizing that their drugs are driving thousands of children crazy, doctors are blaming the problem on the children. As a result, large numbers of children are being diagnosed with bipolar disorder (manic-depressive disorder) when they are really suffering from stimulant and antidepressant drug toxicity.

Drug advocates will go even further in their efforts to hide the truth about the harm that these drugs do to children. The Texas study mentioned above, for example, buried the fact that Prozac caused mania in 6 percent of the children in the clinical trial. The data was hidden in a section on dropouts and was left out of the summary and conclusion. I knew about the finding in advance so I was able to search for it and find it. Even so, it took me time to locate the data.

Based on a preview of the study, I had already challenged the authors of the study to explain how they could consider a drug safe when it caused such a high rate of mania. Emslie, the senior author, declined to respond to my letter when it was published in a psychiatric newspaper.[7]

SSRIs and School Shooters

Eric Harris, the high school senior who perpetrated the mass murders at Columbine High School in Colorado, was taking the SSRI Luvox. Eric had been on the drug for a year while he was developing his violent outlook and plans.[8] A major news magazine claimed that Harris stopped taking his Luvox to let out his anger, but in fact he had an effective level of Luvox in his body at the time of the shooting. I confirmed this information through the Freedom of Information Act that allows any citizen to obtain reports made to the FDA about adverse drug reactions. As required by law, Solvay, the manufacturer of Luvox, sent a report to the FDA about Harris's autopsy. The toxicology report confirmed that Eric had a "therapeutic" or effective level of Luvox in his body at the time of death. Although Eric's name was expunged from the report, it was easy to identify him by the details of the school shooting.

Nor should one be surprised that Luvox can make young people profoundly disturbed and even violent and psychotic. The FDA-approved label for Luvox discloses that 4 percent of children taking the drug for obsessive-compulsive disorder became manic during the ten-week-long controlled clinical trials.[9] By contrast, none of the children who took placebo became manic. An even higher percentage will become manic and psychotic in actual clinical practice where drug monitoring is much more lax and where the drug exposure is much lengthier. Harris, for example, took Luvox for about one year but the 4 percent of young people who became manic on Luvox had taken it for only two and a half months.

Scientific Reports Linking
SSRIs to School Shootings

In Chapter 7 as well as earlier in this chapter, I reviewed studies that link SSRIs to violence in adults and in children. In Chapter 8 I also discussed drug-induced mania and violence. There are additional clinical reports in the literature that specifically link SSRIs to the kind of violence found in school shootings.

In 1999 David Wilkinson, a British psychiatrist, evoked images of school shootings at the start of his clinical presentation of a case in the *Journal of Psychopharmacology*. He described how a previously nonviolent fifteen-year-old boy overturned display stands in a shop, smashed a fellow student in the mouth, and committed a robbery when he was taking Prozac. Wilkinson suggested that this youngster's violence was based more on SSRI-induced emotional blunting than on akathisia.[10] He observed that British psychiatrists are being pressed to give SSRIs to children but that he has not attended any seminars where adverse effects such as akathisia, emotional blunting, and violence have been formally discussed.

In response to Wilkinson's observations, psychiatrist David Healy (1999) pointed out that after the Columbine tragedy the American Psychiatric Association came to the defense of drugs, declaring, "Despite a decade of research, there is little valid evidence to prove a causal relationship between the use of antidepressant medications and destructive behavior."[11] To dispel that myth, Healy refers to his own 1999 review of suicide in association with SSRIs.

I have already cited studies showing how Prozac can make children psychotic, manic, and aggressive. But there's a more dramatic and specific demonstration in the scientific literature concerning its potential to produce a school shooter. King and his colleagues (1991) at Yale University reported on the results of prescribing Prozac to children in clinical trials used for drug research as well as in routine treatment at their clinic. They found that six of forty-two children ages ten to seventeen developed suicidal or violent reactions that seemed clearly related to being put on Prozac.

One of the boys in King's report, a twelve-year-old called Fred,[12] had to be taken out of a controlled clinical trial involving Prozac because of nightmares in which he went to school and killed his classmates. The terrifying dreams were so vivid that Fred began to lose his sense of reality about them. They began to seem real to him. This is how the researchers described Fred's reaction after thirty-eight days on Prozac: "Fred experienced a violent nightmare about killing his classmates until he himself was shot. He awakened from it only with difficulty, and the dream continued to feel 'very real.' He reported having had several days of increasingly vivid 'bad dreams' before this episode; these including images of killing himself and of his parents dying. When he was seen later that day he was agitated and anxious, and refused to go to school."

The Yale researchers removed Fred from Prozac and hospitalized him. Over a period of several weeks he gradually recovered. But his problems didn't end there. He became a victim of the reluctance of doctors to admit that psychiatric drugs can make children emotionally disturbed. When Fred got home from the hospital, his local doctor put him back on Prozac. Fred then became severely suicidal. Once again, he gradually improved after being removed from the drug.

Fred was not having "copycat" nightmares or fantasies. The school shootings had not yet happened. The study was published in 1991 and Fred's experience probably took place a year or two earlier—a long time before the outbreak of school shootings in the late 1990s.

Fred's experience on Prozac actually provides a window into the potential development of a school shooter under the influence of Prozac or any other SSRI. We can easily see how he might have become a school shooter similar to Eric Harris. Fred's antidepressant drug toxicity was discovered and any potential tragedy was averted because he was being carefully supervised and monitored in a controlled clinical trial.

Allowing the Prescription of Unauthorized Drugs to Children

After a drug is FDA-approved for distribution in the United States, the government has little or no control over how doctors choose to prescribe it. Other than to approve or disapprove marketing the drug in the United States and to change its label, the FDA is not allowed to interfere in the actual practice of medicine. Once the drug is put on the market, doctors are free to use the drug in any way they choose.

The only government restraints regularly exercised over the prescribing habits of doctors involve "controlled substances" that are considered addictive and subject to abuse. Stimulants such as Ritalin and Adderall are controlled substances. So are the most powerful barbiturate sedatives, as well as the strongest narcotic painkillers like codeine and morphine. But the SSRIs are not. No agency is looking over the shoulder of doctors to see if they are prescribing these drugs in a dangerous fashion.

A prescription is called "off label" if its use deviates from its approved label. Off-label prescribing can at times be justified in general medical practice. For example, an antibiotic may be approved for one kind of bacterial infection but further research or clinical experiences may show it to be useful against other bacteria.

Although SSRIs like Prozac, Zoloft, Paxil, and Celixa are not approved for the treatment of depression in children, there is no law that prohibits a doctor from prescribing them to depressed children. This freedom to treat may be valuable in other areas of medicine, but in the psychiatric treatment of children, off-label prescribing has become irrational and abusive.

Even if a drug has never been approved for any psychiatric purpose, some doctors will prescribe it for children to control their behavior. For example, clonidine (Catapres) is a drug that is approved for the treatment of hypertension in adults. However, it is very sedating and therefore makes children sleepy and apathetic. I have seen children barely able to stay awake in my office as a result of taking clonidine. Many doctors have taken to prescribing clonidine to counteract the stimulating effects of stimulant and antidepressant drugs, or simply to subdue a difficult youngster.

Doctors are also prescribing unapproved antipsychotic or neuroleptic drugs to children, including Risperdal and Zyprexa. They commonly cause several behavioral abnormalities and can inflict permanent neurological disorders.

Evidence for the Usefulness of SSRIs for Children

Many doctors think that antidepressants can help children, but research indicates that not only are they harmful, they are useless. A 1995 headline in *Clinical Psychiatry News* summed up the current situation: "Though Data Lacking, Antidepressants Used Widely in Children."[13] A 1996 review concluded that no antidepressants "have demonstrated greater efficacy than placebo in alleviating depressive symptoms in children and adolescents."[14] In another review, Seymour and Rhoda Fisher (1996) pointed out that even after admitting that there's no evidence to support giving antidepressants to children, textbooks recommend the practice. They concluded, "The prescribing of antidepressants for children clearly illustrates how a significant group of practitioners (child psychiatrists and pediatricians) can persist in using a procedure that is actually contradicted by research data."

A Situation Entirely Out of Control

Doctors are prescribing extremely dangerous drugs to children for purposes that, in the past, would not have led a doctor to prescribe anything for them. They are exposing children to gigantic risks with little hope of benefit. On top of that, some doctors are prescribing cocktails of three, four, and five drugs at once.

Increased adverse drug effects are inevitable from such a cocktail. Meanwhile, there is not a shred of clinical or scientific evidence to justify the use of multiple psychiatric drugs in treating children. Every one of these children is being subjected to a radical but unsupervised medical experiment.

Forcing Parents to Drug Their Children

I have been a consultant or legal expert in several cases in which schools and even mental hospitals have tried to force parents to drug their child under threat of charging them with medical neglect and removing custody of the child. In other cases, a parent who favors medicating a child has sued in court to gain custody on the grounds that the other parent is against medication. Especially when the child has been grossly overmedicated, I have been able to convince courts or the offending party to give up their attempts to force the parent to go along with medication.

The case of the Weathers family of Millbrook, New York, was a close call. It was covered extensively in the press, and Patricia Weathers joined me in testifying before the Committee on Education and the Workplace of the U.S. House of Representatives in September 2000. Her son Michael had experienced difficulty paying attention and controlling his behavior at school. The school urged the Weathers to have Michael evaluated by a doctor, who immediately prescribed stimulant medication for "ADHD." When Michael got worse, the doctor prescribed Paxil. After that, Michael became extremely anxious and heard voices commanding him to run away. He had violent outbursts for the first time in his life.

Michael's doctor wanted to put him in a mental hospital, but his parents decided that taking him off the Paxil was the wisest choice—and they were right. As they slowly tapered the medication, Michael began a gradual several-week recovery from his drug-induced psychosis.

However, the school psychologist—who was not even a medical doctor—mistakenly concluded that Paxil couldn't cause a child to become disturbed, and he urged the Weathers to put Michael back on psychiatric medication. When they refused, the school reported the Weathers to child protective services for "medical neglect" for refusing to give psychoactive medication to their own child.

The Weathers continued to reject psychiatric medication for Michael. They could see he was improving medication-free while they kept him at home. In the middle of this controversy, they brought him to me for an evaluation.

From the history and from my examination, it was apparent that Michael had never had any serious psychiatric problems until he was put on a stimulant drug. As stimulants often do to children, the drug made Michael depressed. Instead of stopping the medication, the doctor began adding other drugs, including antidepressants. Eventually, Michael ended up on Paxil, the drug that caused a psychotic reaction.

By the time I met Michael several weeks after he was free of Paxil, he was slowly returning to normal and showed no signs whatsoever of being psychotic. He's now doing well in a private school without any medication. He continues to have some problems paying attention and controlling his behavior, but he's never violent, and the school is patient with him as he learns how to enjoy and make the most of school.

Meanwhile, after a visit to their home, child protective services backed down, but the Weathers were subjected to a terrifying and humiliating inquisition. Now they have a permanent record on file indicating that they were charged with child neglect. They also had extensive medical and legal costs to fight the school and child protective services, and now they are paying for a private school.

Tragically, the failure of antidepressants to prove effective for children has been largely ignored by many practicing psychiatrists, pediatricians, and other health professionals. Professionals and parents alike should reject the idea of subjecting any child to SSRIs.

TEN

Withdrawal Problems When Stopping Antidepressants

I've been taking Paxil since it first came out a few years ago, and now I can't get off it. Every time I try to stop, I get nauseated and then I start vomiting. I get terrible headaches, and funny feelings inside my head, and my muscles ache, too. And I get worried that I'll never be able to get off this stuff.

Many people are discovering that although it was easy to start taking SSRI antidepressants, it can be very difficult to stop taking them. Similarly, whereas almost any doctor seems willing to encourage a patient to take these drugs, few doctors know anything about how to withdraw patients from them.

How Drugs Cause Withdrawal Reactions

Any psychoactive drug alters a person's mood by changing the chemistry of brain cells called neurons. These changes cause abnormalities in neuronal functioning. From alcohol and cocaine to

SSRI antidepressants, psychoactive drugs work by creating these disturbances or abnormalities in brain functioning.

The brain itself fights back against these drug-induced abnormalities and this creates additional distortions in the functioning of the brain. As described in earlier chapters, exposure to SSRI antidepressants causes a dieback of receptors for serotonin in the brain.

After the drug is reduced in dosage or stopped, it takes time for the brain to recover. Withdrawal effects show up during the recovery period. They are caused in part by the delay in the brain's return to normal functioning.

An Example from a Non-Prescription Drug

Alcohol is the most commonly used psychoactive drug in our culture. When a person drinks alcohol, the brain becomes sedated or suppressed. If large enough amounts of alcohol are ingested, the brain can become comatose.

But the brain doesn't take this suppression lying down. It fights back. In effect, the brain drives itself into an overexcited or overstimulated condition in its attempt to resist the sedating effects of the alcohol. If the intake of alcohol is abruptly reduced or stopped, the brain for a time will remain overstimulated, resulting in a withdrawal reaction. Depending on the degree of exposure to alcohol and the abruptness of the withdrawal, withdrawal reactions from alcohol occur along a continuum from mild irritability and insomnia to extreme agitation, sleeplessness, and seizures.

Lack of Physician Awareness

Many physicians do not seem aware of how often psychiatric drugs cause withdrawal reactions. In *Your Drug May Be Your Problem: How and Why to Stop Taking Psychiatric Medications* (1999) my coauthor, David Cohen, and I describe how most or all psychiatric drugs can in reality cause withdrawal symptoms, including very dangerous ones.

Lithium, for example, is a toxic element that suppresses over-all brain function and therefore is used to control the occurrence of manic episodes. During the first few weeks or months after stopping lithium, there is an increased risk of developing manic episodes. The individual's risk of mania during lithium with-drawal will be much higher than the individual's previous risk of mania before ever starting the drug.

The so-called antipsychotic drugs, such as Haldol, Zyprexa, and Risperdal, can also cause obvious withdrawal reactions that make it hard for many patients to stop taking them. In some cases, they produce a "withdrawal emergent psychosis." If the psychosis becomes permanent, it is called a "tardive psychosis" to designate that it resulted from exposure to the drugs.[1]

In regard to the stimulant drugs, such as Ritalin and Adderall, studies have shown that even one dose can produce some degree of withdrawal a few hours later. Children who are prescribed these drugs early in the day to suppress their behavior often develop anxiety, agitation, insomnia, and a worsening of their behavior af-ter the drug effect begins to wear off later in the day. However, stimulant withdrawal reactions vary enormously. Some children experience no obvious serious effects when withdrawing from stimulants, but others will "crash" into a state of exhaustion and depression.

Rebound Versus Withdrawal

Rebound is a special kind of withdrawal in which the original symptoms, such as anxiety or depression, become worse than ever before during withdrawal. This chapter has already de-scribed a very dangerous kind of rebound—the increased fre-quency of manic attacks during lithium withdrawal. As a more common example, people frequently experience their most severe and frequent anxiety attacks when they try to stop taking the so-called antianxiety drugs. These drugs, including Xanax, Ativan, Klonopin, and Valium, can cause such severe withdrawal anxiety that patients find themselves unable to stop taking them.

Interdose Withdrawal

If a drug is short-acting, then it can produce withdrawal effects before the next dose is scheduled to be taken. I have already mentioned how a child taking stimulant drugs in the morning or at lunch can undergo withdrawal reactions by the afternoon or evening. Paxil is the most short-acting of the SSRIs and therefore the most likely to produce interdose withdrawal.

Withdrawal from the Older "Tricyclic" Antidepressants

The older tricyclic antidepressants are often designated by their chemical name rather than by their often multiple trade names. They include amitriptyline (Elavil), imipramine (Tofranil), nortriptyline (Pamelor), desimpramine (Norpramin) and clomipramine (Anafranil). It has been known for decades that these antidepressants can have serious withdrawal problems, yet surveys have indicated that many physicians are unaware of the problem.

Typically, people withdrawing from the tricyclic antidepressants will undergo hard-to-describe painful emotions, along with a flulike syndrome with headache, nausea and even vomiting, diarrhea, and aching all over. Insomnia can be troubling, abnormal movements can be disconcerting and painful, and cardiac arrhythmias can be dangerous. The nausea can be especially persistent, and I have consulted with patients who have stayed on these drugs rather than continuing to feel nauseated. These older antidepressants, like the newer SSRIs, can also induce both depression and mania during withdrawal.

Another group of antidepressants, the so-called MAOIs, can also produce severe withdrawal reactions, including depression, mania, abnormal sensations, and psychosis with aggression. These drugs include Nardil, Parnate, and Eldepryl, and in Canada, Manerix.

There is little information about withdrawal problems in regard to most of the newer non-SSRI antidepressants, such as

Wellbutrin or Zyban (buproprion), Serzone (nefazodone), Remeron (mirtazapine), and Desyrel (trazodone). However, doctors and patients should assume that any antidepressant can cause withdrawal reactions, including painful and potentially disabling emotional disturbances.

SSRI Withdrawal Symptoms

I was among the first to warn about SSRI withdrawal reactions in *Talking Back to Prozac* (1994) but now their existence should be common knowledge among physicians. The reactions are caused by the sudden withdrawal of stimulation of the serotonin nervous system. Other drugs that stimulate serotonin, such as Effexor (venlafaxine), can cause withdrawal reactions that are similar to those induced by SSRIs.

Different individuals will experience a wide variation in both the manifestations and the intensity of withdrawal reactions from SSRIs. Although SSRIs most often tend to be stimulating and agitating and to cause insomnia and weight loss, they can also cause sedation and excessive sleep. Similarly, during withdrawal they can cause depression or mania, as well as a variety of other reactions, some people suffering greatly during the process and others relatively little.

The Most Common SSRI Withdrawal Problems

A panel of experts reviewed the commonly reported SSRI withdrawal symptoms.[3] These included dizziness and loss of balance; nausea, vomiting, and other gastrointestinal problems; flulike symptoms of fatigue, muscle aches, and chills; abnormal feelings, such as tingling, burning, or electric shock feelings; and sleep problems, such as insomnia and nightmares.

The panel also found "possibly aggressive and impulsive behavior."[4] Other psychological symptoms of SSRI withdrawal included anxiety or agitation, irritability and dramatic crying spells, depressed mood, and depersonalization. Some patients had problems with slowed thinking, confusion, and memory problems. Some displayed abnormal movements. I have also seen a number of people who experienced severe headaches and other distressing feelings in their heads, including "electrical shocks," as well as abnormal sounds in their ears.

The Most Dangerous
SSRI Withdrawal Reactions

Withdrawal from SSRIs can take two diametrically opposite directions. Some people tend to "crash" into feeling more depressed and even suicidal during the withdrawal, but a smaller number experience mania with an irrational sense of well-being, overexcitation, and poor judgment. As already documented in earlier chapters, both depression and mania can be disastrous for individuals, causing them to take actions that can ruin their lives or the lives of other people. In depression, suicide is the worst outcome. In mania, rash decisions can break off lifetime relationships, cause financial ruin, and even lead to violence.

It's ironic and tragic that these drugs, which people take in the hope of lifting their depression, can cause both depression and mania while they are being taken and during withdrawal from them. The tragedy is compounded when doctors fail to realize that the patient is undergoing a withdrawal reaction, and instead conclude that the patient is suffering from a primary case of worsening depression or mania. The patient may even be put back on the drug, and other drugs may be added to the regimen, when the patient really needs to be withdrawn from the offending drug.

Differences in Withdrawal
Reactions Among SSRIs

As already emphasized, the shorter the drug's duration of action, the more likely that it will tend to cause severe withdrawal reactions. Paxil has the shortest duration of action among the SSRIs. After each dose, the blood level will drop to approximately one-half within a few hours. Withdrawal reactions from Paxil can begin to take place within less than a day.

There are so many reports of severe adverse reactions during withdrawal from Paxil that I have become a medical consultant in a suit against the manufacturer, SmithKline Beecham, on behalf of the citizens of California.

Zoloft, Luvox, and Celexa have longer durations of action than Paxil. Half of each dose may be eliminated from the body in approximately one day. Withdrawal reactions typically occur within the first four days after stopping.

Prozac's duration of action is much longer than Paxil's. It can take a week or more after the last dose for the blood level to fall by one-half. So when people stop taking Prozac abruptly, they are nonetheless withdrawing from the drug at a comparatively slow pace. However, people do experience withdrawal reactions from Prozac, usually starting several days or weeks after terminating the drug. If the person has been taking the medication for several months or more, I recommend a gradual withdrawal.

In my experience, withdrawal reactions from any drug can take longer to develop than suggested by their rate of elimination from the body. Sometimes it can take several weeks for withdrawal symptoms to develop from relatively short-acting drugs. Fatty tissues may be slow to release all of the drug into the bloodstream. The brain may take a while to fully react to the removal of the drug. Also, even a small amount of the drug in the body may somewhat protect against a full-blown withdrawal reaction.

Once a withdrawal reaction begins, there's no accurate way to determine in advance how long it will last. There's considerable variability with withdrawal reactions lasting from one day to as long as several months or more.

The Danger of Irreversible
Withdrawal Reactions

Some patients feel that they have never fully recovered from the effects of antidepressant drugs, suggesting a persistent or chronic withdrawal reaction. However, there are no clinical studies aimed at determining if some people do experience irreversible withdrawal reactions. Until recently, there were no studies of whether the brain itself can recover from drastic SSRI-induced changes, such as the disappearance of serotonin receptors, but recent research has confirmed that some SSRI-induced brain abnormalities can become permanent (Chapter 2).

There are also clinical indications that some patients do not fully recover after the withdrawal process. For example, some patients develop a pathological obesity in response to long-term treatment with SSRIs. This may reflect the failure of the brain to recover from the SSRI receptor dieback.

Anticipating How You
Might React to Withdrawal

In regard to most psychoactive agents, you can anticipate that withdrawal will usually bring about symptoms that are the opposite of the drug's effect on you. Alcohol, antianxiety tranquilizers, and sleeping pills sedate the brain, so the brain compensates by becoming excited, and this stimulation shows up during withdrawal. Ritalin and amphetamines tend to suppress spontaneous behavior of children, leading to a robotic submissiveness, and during withdrawal later in the day, many children become more rambunctious, overactive, and difficult to control.

If antidepressants have tended to sedate or quiet you, then be alert for excitation during withdrawal, whereas if they have tended to stimulate or agitate you, be prepared to feel lethargic or even depressed. However, these guidelines are by no means infallible, and withdrawl reactions can be very unpredictable.

During withdrawal from any psychoactive drug, be prepared for almost any kind of emotional distress or disturbance. The longer you have been taking the drug, the more likely you are to have a serious withdrawal reaction.

How to Handle Withdrawal from SSRIs

The best way to avoid withdrawal is never to take psychoactive drugs for more than a day or two. With some drugs, even a day or two can result in withdrawal reactions.

No drugs have proven useful in helping people withdraw from SSRIs. However, since Prozac has the longest duration of action and hence the potentially most gradual withdrawal, it may at times be useful to switch to Prozac during the withdrawal process from shorter-acting SSRIs.

Because of the unpredictability and potential severity of withdrawal reactions from almost any psychiatric drug, it's important to consult with a professional who knows about the drug before beginning your withdrawal. You probably started taking the SSRI because of emotional problems, such as feelings of depression or obsessions and compulsions, and these may worsen during withdrawal. Especially if you started taking the drug to deal with serious emotional problems, it's a good idea to seek counseling at the same time.

Ten Principles for Withdrawing from Psychiatric Drugs

Here are ten general principles that apply to withdrawing from antidepressants:

First, especially if you have been taking large doses for a long time, find an experienced professional to help you go through the withdrawal process.

Second, if you experienced serious emotional problems before you started taking the drug, be sure to get psychological help before, during, and after the withdrawal process.

Third, tell close family members or friends that you're withdrawing from a psychoactive drug. Explain that withdrawing from antidepressants can cause depression or mania. Ask them to tell you if you start to behave in a manner that's at all worrisome or alarming. *You want others to be watching over you because it's often difficult to be objective about your own behavior during drug withdrawal.*

Fourth, unless you are having a serious adverse drug reaction that requires withdrawing more quickly, go slow, even slower than you think you need to. If you lower the drug dose no faster than 10 percent each week for ten weeks, it will usually help to avoid most serious withdrawal reactions.

Fifth, don't believe your medical doctor if he or she claims that antidepressants don't cause withdrawal problems. Many doctors are ignorant about antidepressant withdrawal reactions.

Sixth, pay attention to how you feel during the withdrawal process except in an emergency under medical supervision, don't reduce the doses any faster than feels comfortable or safe to you. Be alert to a possible drug withdrawal if your mood begins to swing up and down, if you become irritable or angry, if you get odd sensations in your head or skin, if you have trouble sleeping, if your digestive system gets upset, or if your body feels ill.

Seventh, if you start to have what seems like a serious withdrawal reaction, immediately consult with a professional who has clinical experience. At the same time, you might ask your doctor about resuming your previous dose—the one you were taking just before your last reduction. If you are having a withdrawal reaction, returning to the previous higher dose will usually provide rapid relief.

Eighth, if you are trying to withdraw from several psychiatric drugs, it's generally best to withdraw from one at a time. Withdrawing from two or more drugs at once can be confusing. If you begin to have a withdrawal reaction, you may not be able to figure out which drug is the culprit. In complex situations involving several drugs, you and your doctor may benefit from reading *Your Drug May Be Your Problem: How and Why to Stop Taking Psychiatric Medications* by me and David Cohen.

Ninth, it's not uncommon to run into a stubborn withdrawal reaction while trying to taper off the very last dose of the drug. Some of my patients have found it helpful to take tiny amounts of the drug—small fractions of the smallest recommended dose—to ward off the last vestiges of the withdrawal reaction.

Keep in mind that my observations and suggestions are not intended to provide a complete guideline to withdrawing from SSRIs or any other psychiatric drugs. I urge people to get support from a trusted, experienced professional, as well as from family and friends, when going through a potentially difficult drug withdrawal.

ELEVEN

Physical Conditions That Cause or Worsen Depression

In a typical private practice of psychotherapy, medicine, or psychiatry, most depressed patients are suffering from obvious psychological causes, such as loss of a loved one or a job, or other pressures at home or work. However, people can also become depressed as a result of a variety of physical illnesses and physical stressors. Unfortunately, doctors who believe in the mythical "biochemical imbalance" will too often overlook the possibility of a more genuine physical cause for their patient's depression, such as thyroid dysfunction or psychiatric drug intoxication.

Generally we speak of two "schools of thought" about the cause of depression. One school is considered "psychological" and the other "biological," but the distinction can be very confusing and even misleading. For example, although I believe that most cases of depression originate from relatively obvious psychological and social stresses, on occasion I find that patients are depressed in part by undiagnosed physical diseases. Sometimes biologically oriented psychiatrists have failed to suspect the physical ailment. In their zeal to believe that their patients have "biochemical imbalances," these doctors can overlook obvious physical causes, including the psychiatric drugs that they are prescribing to their patients.

This chapter aims at alerting patients and practitioners to the array of genuine physical disorders—in contrast to "biochemical imbalances"—that can cause or contribute to feelings of depression.

The Elusive Biochemical Imbalance

The huge economic resources of the psychopharmaceutical industry, the might of the federal government, and the authority of the medical profession back this biochemical model of depression. However, might has never made right, and there's little or no evidence for this biological viewpoint. Even biologically oriented textbooks of psychiatry end up admitting that there's no convincing proof that depression or manic-depressive (bipolar) disorder is genetic or physical in origin. A "scientific breakthrough" is always imminent but somehow never materializes.

Science does not possess the technology to measure biochemical imbalances in the living brain. The "biochemical imbalances" speculation is actually a drug company–sponsored marketing campaign to sell drugs. The speculation has also been promoted as truth by biological psychiatrists to convince patients to come to them rather than to nonmedical therapists.

Ironically, it is certain that psychiatric drugs cause biochemical imbalances in the brain, but drug advocates claim that these imbalances are advantageous to the patient.

Whether there are genetic factors that cause or contribute to depression is also a scientific question, and science has not confirmed any genetic basis for the depresion or manic-depressive disorder.

Meanwhile, there's a great deal of scientific evidence to confirm that people become depressed because of their life experiences. In particular, childhood experiences such as abandonment, abuse, and neglect can lead to depression. Adult experiences of trauma and loss also can cause depression.[1]

We can also utilize self-knowledge about our own emotions. We have firsthand experience with only one life—our own. How do we experience the origins of our feelings? Do we become depressed completely out of the blue, or do we become depressed because we lost a loved one, became overwhelmed with the stresses of life, or faced repeated disappointments in our love or work lives?

I have examined the psychological causes of depression in chapter 1 and will return to the subject in the final chapter of the book, which focuses on how to overcome depression.

Physical Disorders that Can Cause Depression

Although biochemical balances remain in the realm of sheer speculation, there are a variety of physical disorders and stressors that can make people feel depressed.

When people become physically ill from almost any cause, they can lapse into feeling despair and helplessness. But what's causing the depressed feelings—a primary effect on the brain or the person's psychological reaction to being ill? The answer is uncertain. Whatever the ultimate cause many physical conditions make people vulnerable to becoming depressed.

If we think about their physical effects, it's no wonder that people at times become depressed in response to hormonal disorders such as hypothyroidism and diabetes, viral disorders such as infectious mononucleosis and hepatitis, or neurological diseases such as multiple sclerosis and Parkinsonism. Each of these disorders can impair our mental faculties, undermine our sense of overall wellness, limit our energy and our activities, make us feel helpless and dependent, and confront us with our mortality. The chronic loss of energy associated with these disorders would in itself lead many people to feel, at the least, seriously discouraged. It takes an especially positive attitude toward adversity to remain relatively cheerful and hopeful in the face of these stresses.

Because the underlying problem is at least in part psychological, people with stressful, debilitating diseases can often find inspiration from loved ones, self-help groups, religion, or therapy. Their spirits can often be lifted by a viewpoint that enables them to overcome their sense of psychological helplessness. Often they do this by finding meaning in their suffering, especially by using their suffering to reach out to others in need.

Medications as the Cause of Depressed Feelings

Medications are at the top of the list of physical factors that make people vulnerable to becoming depressed. In particular, almost any drug that disrupts the biochemistry of the brain is likely to make some people feel depressed.

I've already described how antidepressants often worsen depression. I also mentioned the extreme example of Rebetron, the medication used to treat hepatitis C. I noted that the 1990 *Health Letter* listed more than a dozen types of medications that cause depression and that the 1998 *Medical Letter* named more than 100 categories of medications and individual drugs that produce psychiatric reactions. The consensus in the medical community is that many medications can cause or make people vulnerable to serious emotional or psychiatric problems.

Psychiatric Drugs Known to Cause or Worsen Depression

The list of psychiatric drugs that can drive a person toward depression is extensive and includes the following:

Antidepressants, including SSRIs like Prozac, Paxil, Zoloft, Celexa, and Luvox.

Stimulant drugs, such as Ritalin, Metadate, Concerta, Dexedrine, and Adderall. It seems counterintuitive that stimulants could cause depression and even doctors don't know that depression commonly results from taking these chemical agents. Many children are initially given stimulants for minor school or behavioral problems, and then develop drug-induced depression, leading to antidepressant therapy and a progressive worsening of their mental condition.

"Antianxiety drugs," tranquilizers, and sleeping medications, especially the benzodiazepines, including Xanax (alprazolam), Halcion (triazolam), Ativan (lorazepam), Klonopin (clonazepam), Librium (chlordiazepoxide), and Valium (diazepam). Benzodiazepines are very addictive, and they cause anxiety, insomnia, headache, and muscle spasms during regular treatment but even more so when people try to withdraw from them. As a result, many people remain on them for months and years at a time, and end up chronically depressed and anxious as a result of the drug effects. However, the patients rarely realize that the drugs are depressing them and, unfortunately, their doctors often diagnose their depression as a psychiatric disorder rather than as a drug reaction.

"Mood stabilizers" such as lithium and Depakote (divalproex). One of my patients, an active woman in her thirties, had been put on lithium by her HMO, Kaiser Permanente, and became chronically depressed. She lost her interest in work and in her social life, and withdrew into living in her mother's home. Eventually routine blood chemistry tests showed that the lithium had caused her irreversible kidney disease, and at that point, after too long a delay, she was taken off the drug. Her mood immediately improved, and after reading one of my books, she realized that she'd been living in a paralyzing depression that was caused by the lithium. She asked me to be her doctor and then her medical

expert. She sued Kaiser for improperly prescribing and supervising her lithium treatment, and received a six-figure settlement.

Neuroleptics (also called "antipsychotics") such as Risperdal (risperidone), Zyprexa (olanzapine), Seroquel (quetiapine), Clozaril (clozapine), Haldol (haloperidol), and Prolixin (fluphenazine). Another of my patients, a bright graduate student in her late twenties, became so stupefied and depressed on Zyprexa that she was unable to pursue her studies. The drug blunted her mind to the extent that she was unable to appreciate what was happening to her, but her psychiatrist insisted that she "needed" the drug. She began to look like a "zombie" and worried family members brought her to me for a consultation. She entered treatment with me for the purpose of withdrawing from her drugs, as well as for longer-term psychotherapy. After she got through a difficult withdrawal period, she realized that Zyprexa had been depressing her to the point of emotional paralysis. She was able to return to school.

Recreational Drugs That
Can Cause Depression

Chronic alcohol use can cause people to feel depressed without their appreciating it. Marijuana will also have this effect in such a subtle fashion that the drug users have no idea how apathetic or "blue" they have become. From Ritalin (see above) to Ecstasy, stimulants can also end up producing depression.

Medical Disorders That
Commonly Cause Depression

Earlier I mentioned that numerous medical disorders can cause or contribute to depressed feelings. The following is a partial list:

Hormonal disorders, such as hypothyroidism, estrogen imbalances caused by menopause or by surgical removal of the ovaries, diabetes, and Cushing's disease. Doctors are too prone to prescribe psychiatric medication to women without referring them for medical evaluation for treatable hormonal problems. Sometimes the women are already receiving hormonal replacement and the psychiatrist mistakenly assumes that the hormonal therapy is being properly conducted, when the dose or type of hormone is inappropriate. In some instances, I've seen patients whose previous psychiatrists have failed to take even a brief medical history that would have disclosed signs of hypothyroidism, such as weight gain, cold intolerance, dry skin, and hair loss.

Viral disorders, including hepatitis and mononucleosis. Anyone suffering infectious hepatitis or mononucleosis is likely to feel depressed, often without realizing that the depression results from being physically ill. After doing poorly in her first two months of college, a young woman was hospitalized for hepatitis. No one told her that her difficulty in studying was probably related to the developing viral disease, and so she felt like a failure. As a result, she became depressed and dropped out of school.

Chronic Fatigue Syndrome, fibromyalgia, rheumatoid arthritis, lupus erythematosus, and related autoimmune disorders. Many immune disorders, some of them controversial in nature, first appear as chronic fatigue. Like any disorders that produce tiredness and exhaustion, depression can also be the first sign of the disease. Too often these patients are put on psychiatric drugs that complicate their problems, and can even worsen their disorders by further compromising the immune system and brain function.

Neurological disorders such as Alzheimer's, Parkinsonism, multiple sclerosis, and Huntington's chorea. Four decades ago in medical school I was taught that depression can become the first sign of a brain tumor or other neurological disorders. But the lesson is often lost on modern psychiatrists, who are too ready to blame mythological biochemical imbalances, overlooking the possibility of real disease.

Cancer, AIDS, and other debilitating disorders. Any disorder that exhausts the body or threatens life can also deplete the spirit. Too often these people are given psychiatric drugs instead of counseling to help them cope with and even triumph over their feelings of fear and despair.

Insomnia from any cause. Insomnia often has a very depressing effect on people. The depression can stem from the underlying cause of the insomnia, such as emotional stress or psychoactive drugs, or it can be a direct effect of disrupted dream life, lost sleep, and resultant fatigue. Individuals who work irregular hours need to be aware of the emotional impact caused by disrupted sleep cycles.

Brain damage from any cause. Both gross and subtle forms of brain damage can cause depression. Closed-head injuries that result from whiplash or falls may at first seem relatively harmless but can produce subtle difficulties in thinking and memory function, as well as emotional instability. Electroshock treatment causes brain damage and, in my clinical experience, can cause lasting depression.

Chronic pain and physical disability. Physical disability frequently causes people to feel hopeless and despairing. The inability to work or to carry out previous recreational activities can lead to depression. Chronic pain obviously makes it harder for the individual to remain optimistic. Too often, these patients are prescribed multiple analgesics and psychiatric medications that worsen their brain function and mental outlook. I've been a treating physician or medical expert in several cases that had progressed from back pain to drug addiction and on to abnormal and even violent behavior. Inspired counseling and proper rehabilitation can often help these individuals have worthwhile, satisfying lives without their succumbing to drug intoxication.

The Importance of a
Good Medical Evaluation

If you've been feeling depressed for more than a few days or weeks, you should have a thorough physical evaluation, including a broad range of blood chemistry studies. Be especially careful that your medical doctor doesn't dismiss the possibility of a physical cause. Physicians have been so indoctrinated by drug company sales representatives, they may offer you an antidepressant rather than a thorough physical workup if you mention anything about feeling depressed.

Even if you think you know why you're depressed—for example, by the loss of a loved one—it remains important to obtain a medical evaluation. Physical causes can combine with environmental stressors to make us especially vulnerable to persistent feelings of depression.

Emotional stress, including depressed feelings, can also cause or worsen physical disorders, so that you can end up both emotionally distressed and physically ill. For example, your sadness may have led you to pay less close attention to your diet, and poor eating can worsen many diseases, including diabetes and a variety of gastrointestinal problems. Poor diet can also lead to increased weakness and fatigue.

Feeling depressed leads to self-neglect. Perhaps your mother became depressed after the death of your father and then stopped taking her medications properly, causing her health to deteriorate. Or perhaps her sadness at his loss led her to ignore the warning pains of an illness such as heart disease.

Diet and Depression

Many "natural therapies" are offered for the cure of depression on the justification that the unhappy feelings are caused by nutritional deficiencies. However, I haven't been impressed by the scientific basis for these claims. Many depressed people are being hoodwinked into spending money for useless dietary supplements. I'm in favor of eating well and taking a good multivitamin as general health measures, but I'm not in favor of loading up on specific dietary supplements as an approach to healing specific emotional problems.

Poor health can make us vulnerable to feeling depressed and anxious. So can a sedentary, mentally inactive life. Conversely, good health and a life of vigorous mental and physical activity help to protect us against feeling helpless, tense, and despairing. Regardless of whether we have a tendency to suffer from depression, we should do everything we can to stay healthy by getting sufficient sleep and exercise, and by creating a life full of interest and challenge.

In fact, new research has shown that exercise is at least as good as SSRI antidepressants in treating depression and has more lasting effects than antidepressants when the patients are evaluated after ten months.[2] Of course, in addition to helping us to overcome depression, exercise brings many additional benefits not associated with taking mind-altering drugs. Exercise improves our physical health and longevity, encourages weight loss, enhances our physical appearance, adds energy to our daily activities, improves sleep, and can bring the pleasure of engaging us with other human beings or with the outdoors and nature. By contrast, psychoactive pill-taking tends to be an isolated activity that often results in severe adverse physical, mental, and social effects.

TWELVE

No Such Thing
As an Antidepressant

Is it possible that there's no such thing as a genuine antidepressant? Before the scientific data had confirmed my suspicions, I doubted that a drug could actually "treat depression." After all, if depression is a product of our conflicts, stressful life experiences, and stifled choices, a drug would have no direct effect on it.

Meanwhile, study after study has confirmed that antidepressants typically perform only a little better than sugar pills. In some studies, antidepressants actually turn out to be less effective than the lowly sugar pill.

Reviewing All the Recent FDA Studies

A group of researchers obtained FDA clinical data from forty-five studies involving seven antidepressants approved from 1987 through 1997, including Prozac and Zoloft.[1] The clinical trials lasted the usual four to six weeks and compared the new drugs with placebo and older antidepressants. Depression "declined" in 41 percent with the newer antidepressants such as the SSRIs, 42 percent with older antidepressants, and 31 percent with placebo. Overall, less than half of the patients in drug-treated groups improved at all. More striking, they only improved 10 percent more than the placebo group, which improved 31 percent.

Meanwhile, so few depressed patients actually recover during antidepressant therapy that the drug companies don't try to measure recovery. Instead, they measure improvement, usually on the basis of a checklist of items filled out during a brief interview with the patient conducted by prodrug researchers.

The lessons from all this are more profound than meet the eye. Not only is the sugar pill almost as good as the antidepressant, it is probably much better. First of all, placebo pills don't produce life-threatening illnesses, psychoses, and aggression. Second, these trials were paid for, designed, and evaluated by the drug companies themselves. Yet the companies couldn't skew them enough to make the antidepressants look anything but marginally effective. Overall, the results suggest that placebo is actually much better than an antidepressant.

Drug Company Tricks

Drug companies try to do everything they can to "get around" the placebo effect. Eli Lilly and Co. was a leading participant in a recent drug company conference aimed solely at how to overcome the embarrassing fact that patients taking placebo often do as well or better than patients taking antidepressants.

A common trick used in contemporary drug research is called the placebo washout. All the participants are put on placebo before they are entered into the actual clinical trials. Any subjects who do particularly well on placebo are then thrown out before the study begins. The modified group of patients—absent those most likely to respond positively to placebo—are then used for the clinical trials that compare the drug to placebo.

By ridding the study of people who respond especially well to placebo, the drug companies skew the data in favor of the drug. This is done in every study I have seen used for FDA approval of antidepressants. The routine use of the placebo washout shows that the FDA and the scientific community will go along with tricks aimed at giving drugs a false image of effectiveness.

Remember that a prodrug review of all antidepressant drug trials used for FDA approval over a ten-year period showed only a 10 percent higher improvement rate compared to placebo. Now imagine if those studies had not used the ubiquitous placebo washout trick. It is extremely likely that the 10 percent difference would have evaporated. The dangerous antidepressants would have proven themselves no more helpful—but a lot more harmful—than the sugar pill.

More Evidence That Antidepressants Do Not Work

Many researchers have explored the failure of antidepressants to prove themselves effective in controlled clinical trials. In fact, even the minimal 10 percent advantage found in the overview of all antidepressant trials used for FDA approval is probably an artifact.

When a drug that has side effects is compared with a sugar pill with no side effects, the drug has a decided advantage in any controlled clinical trial. First, the doctors who are conducting the study can tell by the side effects which patients are taking the "real thing." For example, patients taking Prozac are much more likely to report insomnia, weight loss, and agitation than patients taking a placebo. In other words, the double-blind is broken; the doctor can figure who is getting the antidepressant and who is getting the sugar pill. Therefore, the doctors' bias in favor of the drug comes into play and the drug company–hired doctors who perform these studies are very biased in favor of the drug.

Second, when a drug has noticeable side effects, patients tend to report a greater therapeutic effect. It's the old "snake oil principle" that something that tastes bad must being having a powerful effect. Since depression is an emotional state that often responds well to any encouragement or hope, the experience of mild to moderate adverse effects is likely to add to the drug's "power."

Consistent with what I'm saying, researchers have found that antidepressants do not perform any better in clinical trials than placebo pills that have side effects of their own that are discernable by the doctor and/or the patient. Thus, an active placebo—for example, one that causes dry mouth or sweating—is likely to be rated by patients as doing as much good as an antidepressant.

The observations I'm making are based on both a rational, commonsense analysis of what goes on during a clinical trial and on scientific analyses of clinical trials.[2] They contradict the public relations image of antidepressant therapy as based on science. In fact, antidepressant therapy has very little scientific foundation. Instead, it requires a great deal of manipulation to maintain the misleading viewpoint that antidepressants are effective.

Growing Recognition of Drug Company Influence

The conservative *New England Journal of Medicine* recently published a "Health Policy Report" that challenged what it called the "Uneasy Alliance" between pharmaceutical companies and the clinical investigators that they hire to carry out controlled clinical trials. The article by Thomas Bodenheimer, M.D., in the May 18, 2000, issue of the journal documented how drug company funding skews the results of clinical trials. Drug companies won't support a clinical trial proposal if they suspect that the results won't favor the drug. They retain the right to stop publication of the results when the data do not make the drug look good.

Many drug companies don't let the clinical investigators analyze the data. Instead, they use corporate employees to carry out the analysis clandestinely at the company. This has enabled a corporation like Eli Lilly and Co. to withhold its own reports from the FDA and the profession if they cast any doubt on the drug.

For the reader who wishes to learn more about how drug companies influence everything from scientific research to government policy, I have investigated the problem in a number of my publications, including *Talking Back to Prozac* (1994), *Brain-Disabling Treatments in Psychiatry* (1997), *The War Against Children of Color* (1998), and *Talking Back to Ritalin* (1998, revised in 2001). The data in *Talking Back to Ritalin* was sufficient to inspire the current series of class action suits being brought against Novartis, the manufacturer of Ritalin.[3]

The Myth That Drugs Are Tested on Thousands of People Before They Are Approved

I found estimates by drug advocates that Prozac had been tested on 10,000 people before it was approved. I then went to a great deal of trouble to count the total number of patients who finished the controlled clinical trials for the FDA approval of Prozac. The total turned out to be 286 patients—a far cry from the thousands that most people imagine. In deposing me and in crossexamining me in court, Eli Lilly and Co. has never challenged this figure.

Even the total of 286 is deceiving. Many of the clinical trials are very small with only one or two dozen patients finishing them. As a result, the individual doctor is looking at a very small pool of patients. With such a limited number of patients to look at, the doctor can easily fail to see an emerging pattern of adverse effects and can easily dismiss a possible harmful effect as unrelated to the drug.

The Myth That Millions of Users Are Living Proof of a Drug's Efficacy

The widespread use of Prozac and other SSRI antidepressants might seem to indicate that they are medically useful, emotionally helpful, or otherwise of genuine value. But consider other widely used psychoactive drugs: alcohol, nicotine, marijuana, cocaine, Ecstasy, and heroin. Despite cultural ostracism, legal constraints, great expense, well-known health hazards, condemnation by medical experts, and highly organized antidrug advertising campaigns by the government and by private nonprofit groups—many individuals continue to risk their health and even their lives to take these recreational and illegal drugs. Is it any wonder that people also rush to take legal drugs when their use is *highly promoted* by cultural values, medical experts, prodrug advertising campaigns, the government, and private nonprofit organizations?

When it is understood that SSRIs most closely resemble stimulant drugs such as amphetamine, methamphetamine, Ecstasy, and cocaine in most of their clinical effects, it becomes even easier to understand why millions of people end up taking them. For many people, SSRIs have become legalized stimulants.

SSRIs as Panacea

Prozac was FDA-approved for the treatment of depression in December 1987. Since then it has also been approved for obsessive-compulsive disorder, bulimia nervosa (binge-eating and vomiting), and most recently for premenstrual dysphoric disorder, better known as PMS.

Without necessarily advocating them, one commonly used textbook lists many off-label (not FDA-approved) uses for Prozac, including alcoholism, anorexia nervosa, ADHD, bipolar disorder, borderline personality disorder, narcolepsy (inappropriate falling asleep), kleptomania (compulsive stealing), migraine and tension headaches, posttraumatic stress disorder, syncope (fainting), schizophrenia, social phobia, Tourette's syndrome (tics and vocalizations), and trichotillomania (pulling out hair).

The above list should be taken as a testimonial to the willingness of doctors to prescribe psychoactive agents for almost any condition including those it is much more likely to worsen. Indeed, Prozac is probably more likely to worsen each of those disorders than to improve them.

Starting at the beginning of the list, Prozac can worsen alcoholism by causing agitation, anxiety, insomnia, and other kinds of stimulation that the individual attempts to treat by drinking alcohol. In regard to anorexia nervosa, Prozac commonly causes anorexia and weight loss. In regard to ADHD, Prozac frequently causes hyperactivity in the form of akathisia and agitation. Concerning its use in treating bipolar or manic-depressive disorder, Prozac is known to cause mania. Borderline personality is characterized by difficulty in making relationships, and Prozac tends to render people less able to relate. Narcolepsy might be "helped" by Prozac's tendency to cause insomnia and overstimulation, but it might be worsened by Prozac's contradictory tendency to cause somnolence in some people. Instead of curing kleptomania, Prozac can cause impulsive acts like irrational stealing. And so on . . .

Paxil was approved by the FDA for depression in December 1992. Since then it has also been approved for obsessive-compulsive disorder, panic disorder, and social anxiety disorder. Ironically, all of the SSRIs, including Paxil, are known to cause anxiety. The approval of these drugs to treat anxiety-related conditions is a tribute to the art of conducting controlled clinical trials.

Zoloft was approved for depression in December 1991. I found internal FDA documents in which the head of the division that approves psychiatric drugs was expressing doubt about Zoloft's efficacy on the day of its approval.[4] Zoloft has also been FDA-approved for obsessive-compulsive disorder and panic disorder.

Luvox was FDA-approved for the treatment of obsessive-compulsive disorder in December 1994. It was approved for children as well as adults, but the clinical trials showed a 4 percent rate of mania as an adverse drug effect in children and teenagers. However, its FDA approval for OCD in children has led some doctors to use it as an antidepressant for children.

Celexa was FDA-approved on July 24, 1998, for the treatment of depression. Unfortunately, it is likely to be used for many of the same absurd and dangerous purposes for which Prozac and the other SSRIs are too often used.

SSRIs have also been used for the treatment of obesity. However, this use has been discouraged by the failure of Prozac to gain FDA approval for this purpose, and the recognition that longer-term use of Prozac can lead to pathological obesity.

SSRIs are also commonly used for a variety of pain syndromes, especially headache, but they can also cause headaches. In addition, by making people more anxious and irritable, SSRIs can make patients feel more upset by their pain.

Although the SSRIs have been viewed as panaceas, they aren't even good antidepressants. Their approval for a wide variety of disorders is a testimonial to the craft or craftiness of clinical trial design and evaluation, as well as a commentary on the general tendency of these drugs to anesthetize feelings of any kind and to produce an artificial euphoria in some people.

The Limits of FDA Approval

FDA approval by no means indicates that a drug is truly effective. In fact, psychiatric drugs often are approved on the basis of very marginal evidence for their effectiveness. In *Talking Back to Prozac,* I showed how the FDA approved Prozac despite the fact that the drug was no better than placebo and less effective than the older antidepressants.

When it came time to approve Prozac, the combined efforts of the drug company and the FDA could not come up with even one good study that unequivocally supported the value of Prozac in comparison to placebo. The FDA then decided to break its own rules. It gave approval to Prozac based on its marginal effectiveness *when in combination with addictive tranquilizing drugs that reduced the patients' Prozac-induced agitation, anxiety, and insomnia.* In the end, Prozac was in reality approved as a combination drug—Prozac plus sedative, addictive tranquilizers, such as Valium and Dalmane. But the medical profession and the public were never told.

Even with the illegal addition of tranquilizers to help calm down many Prozac patients, the patients continued to drop out of the FDA studies in large numbers because of adverse Prozac effects. As a result, the FDA had to let Eli Lilly and Co. count patients who dropped out as if they had remained in the study.

I am not alone in finding that there is little evidence for a specific antidepressant effect and that antidepressant drugs have little or no therapeutic advantage over a sugar pill.[5] On the other hand, these drugs do have psychoactive effects. They cause brain dysfunction that either blunts the emotions or causes an artificial euphoria. These stimulantlike effects will give temporary relief to some people when they are suffering from depression or other painful feelings, but in the long run the drugs do more harm than good.

THIRTEEN

From Lobotomy to Electroshock and Brain Stimulation

Many people think that lobotomy and electroshock are "things from the past"—relics of a bygone era in psychiatry. Unfortunately, that's anything but true. Depressed people who feel overwhelmed and desperate for help are frequently subjected to shock treatment and a small number fall victim to newer forms of lobotomy.

Electroshock (also called electroconvulsive therapy, or ECT) has been on the upswing for two decades. Many psychiatric wards in general hospitals and most private mental hospitals have shock rooms where—on Monday, Wednesday, and Friday morning of each week–several patients are sent into convulsions by jolts of electricity sufficient to stop a heart. Although no accurate numbers are available, probably well over 100,000 people each year in the United States are subjected to shock, usually for depression.

Some doctors advocate shock as the first approach to treating depression in the elderly. They believe it's a better alternative than antidepressants because the drugs often cause potentially fatal reactions in the elderly. However, as this chapter will document, the fragile brains of the elderly are easily injured when subjected to the passage of a current the equivalent of a 100-watt bulb going off for a second or two in the brain. Also, there's good evidence that exercise is even a better alternative than drugs for helping older patients overcome depression.[1]

Electric shock treatment was first inflicted on a patient in 1938 in Italy, a scant two years after the first modern lobotomies were inflicted on patients in Portugal in 1936. The patients were involuntary and often protested and even fought to resist the treatment.

The almost simultaneous development of electric shock and lobotomy was no coincidence. Doctors in the mid-1930s were searching for more efficient ways to damage the brain because it made patients manageable during their confinement to the giant public lockups called state mental hospitals. Like the advocates of lobotomy, the shock doctors noticed that the "treatments" rendered inmates quieter, less emotionally spontaneous, and more docile. This made it much easier to run these vast psychiatric prisons under their inhumane and brutal conditions.

Lobotomy and electroshock have similar effects because they both damage the highest evolutionary centers of the human brain, the frontal lobes. In old-fashioned lobotomy, a large scalpel was swished around the underside of the frontal lobes to cut off the connections into the remainder of the brain. Nowadays electrodes are inserted through holes in the skull. Then they are heated up to "cook" brain tissue in or adjacent to the frontal lobes.

Psychosurgery works, and can only work, by so damaging the brain that the individual is no longer able to feel or at least to express the same degree of emotional pain and suffering. Instead, the brain-damaged person becomes relatively numb, docile, and helpless. Inevitably, higher mental functions such as judgment and moral sensitivity are impaired.

If people are surprised that electroshock is growing in popularity, they are even more dismayed that psychosurgery is still being done at all. Again like electroshock, psychosurgery was resurging in the early 1970s, and seemed destined to make a major comeback, until I devoted several years of my professional life to stopping it.

The following story of my campaign to stop psychosurgery illustrates the willingness of psychiatry to defend its treatments no matter how obviously damaging to the brain. It provides the reader a partial answer to the nagging question, "How can psychiatry ignore the brain-damaging effects of antidepressants and other drugs?" The answer is simple: Damaging the brain to impair brain function lies at the heart of *all* the physical treatments in psychiatry. Shock and lobotomy are merely the most egregious examples. I have described this phenomenon as the brain-disabling principle of psychiatric treatment.[2]

Stopping Psychosurgery
on Little Children

My career of reform work as a psychiatrist began in 1972 when I organized an international campaign to stop the return of lobotomy and other forms of psychosurgery. I was especially outraged by experiments being conducted at the University of Mississippi in Jackson in a segregated institution for emotionally distressed and abandoned African-American children. O. J. Andy, the director of neurosurgery at the university, was implanting multiple electrodes in the brains of children as young as five. He would conduct stimulation experiments and then heat the electrodes to destroy various parts of the children's brains. As a serial psychosurgeon, sometimes he would repeat these mutilating experiments several times over a period of months or years. In one case, his own publications showed a decline and deterioration in the child's mental life.

Although most psychosurgery was being conducted on adults, the medical abuse of children particularly appalled me. Although Dr. Andy was publishing his studies at conferences and in journals, no one challenged him—or any of the other psychosurgeons—until I took a public and professional stand.

Taking on the Harvard Surgeons

During the same period of time, Harvard Medical School professors, including neurosurgeons Vernon Mark and William Sweet, were carrying out a project that was made infamous by my campaign to stop psychosurgery. As the head of neurosurgery at the famed Massachusetts General Hospital, Sweet was one of the most respected and powerful men in American medicine. With grants from the National Institute of Mental Health and the Justice Department, the doctors were implanting a shish kebab of dozens of electrodes through the brains of patients for the supposed cure of violence.

Mark and Ervin had obtained their federal support by claiming in writing and in testimony that black urban rioters had brain disease that could be cured by their surgery. At that time, during the late 1960s and early 1970s, the nation was terrified by the specter of these urban disasters, so the government supported racially motivated experiments in psychosurgery.

Because of the racist implications of both the Mississippi and the Boston projects, I was strongly supported in my antipsychosurgery by the Black Caucus of the U.S. Congress. I also drew support from feminists who understood that most psychosurgery, like most shock treatment, is in fact inflicted on women.

Still other psychosurgery projects were being conducted at the National Institutes of Health, the Veterans' Administration, various state hospitals, and a few other university medical centers.

By exposing the surgeons to public humiliation, participating in lawsuits against them, working with a few concerned members of the U.S. Congress, and successfully lobbying for the formation of a psychosurgery commission—my volunteer campaign led to the termination of all of the projects I have described, including those at Harvard and at the University of Mississippi.

The attempted resurgence of psychosurgery was aborted and I was now full steam ahead as a psychiatric reformer. I have continued in that role to this day.

The impact of my reform work persists. As recently as 1992, the Departments of Psychiatry and Neurosurgery at Johns Hopkins Medical School expressed resentment about my thwarting their continued desire to resume psychosurgery. Donlin Long, M.D., chief of neurosurgery, complained that to start performing psychosurgery again he and his colleagues would need "the guts to tell the Peter Breggins of the world to stuff it."[3]

Unfortunately, a few medical centers continue, to this day, to carry out psychosurgery. Currently, for example, I'm a medical expert against a psychosurgeon who disabled a woman during surgery at a famous clinic. At present, psychosurgeons try to claim they are doing it as a routine treatment rather than as the radical, dangerous experiment that it is. Most of the patients are diagnosed with obsessive-compulsive disorder but depressed people also fall victim.

Deep Brain Stimulation

Deep brain stimulation is closely related to psychosurgery. In fact, psychosurgeons like Vernon Mark and O. J. Andy used their implanted electrodes to stimulate various parts of the brain before destroying them by heating up the tip of the inserted electrode. Deep brain stimulation has been used to treat Parkinsonism and now it is being advocated for "mood disorders" and also "anxiety, psychosis, obsessive-compulsive disorder, and Tourette's syndrome."[4] Patients are being trained to stimulate themselves from portable stimulation machines.

Stimulating the brain can cause a wide variety of painful emotions and occasional euphoria, but its potential as a "treatment" is limited by at least two factors. Deep brain stimulation is bound to cause serious harm to the surrounding brain tissue, neuronal function, or both, and it makes no rational sense as a psychiatric treatment. To electronically stimulate oneself with a portable device to cause euphoria seems like the epitome of treating oneself as a "thing" rather than a human being.

Causing Insanity

One of the patients in the experiments conducted by Vernon Mark and William Sweet was a man named Thomas R. During my campaign to stop their surgery, Thomas's mother contacted me. In their publications, Mark and Sweet, along with Harvard psychiatrist Frank Ervin, claimed that their surgery had cured Thomas of his violence without producing any serious side effects. When Mark was forced to release Thomas's medical records to me, and after I met Thomas, it became clear that the doctors had literally driven Thomas mad through the combined effects of brain stimulation and melting brain tissue.

Before the surgery, Thomas was a working engineer whose only violence involved throwing something without striking anyone during a marital quarrel. He underwent the surgery in part to please his wife who nonetheless divorced him during the course of the operations. Even after the electrodes were implanted, Thomas resisted the idea of letting the surgeons melt portions of his brain. According to their own writings, he protested aggressively, until his brain was stimulated into a state of euphoria, at which time he consented to the surgery. This, of course, was highly unethical conduct by the doctors.

The surgery reduced Thomas to a chronic, demented state hospital patient. Later on, he was sometimes mistaken for a "schizophrenic" because he persisted in his "delusional" fear that he was under the control of doctors who could stimulate his brain by remote control, much as they had done on the hospital ward.[5]

Brain stimulation and brain psychosurgery as psychiatric treatments should be considered too experimental and potentially dangerous to be carried out on human subjects.

Trying to Stop
Shock Treatment

When I organized the opposition to psychosurgery in the early 1970s, few professionals dared to join me in standing up to some of the most powerful surgeons, psychiatrists, and medical organizations in the world. However, in recent years many professionals have voiced their opposition to shock treatment. Nonetheless, the treatment is so entrenched within psychiatry that our efforts have hardly dented its revival.

Electrical Closed-Head Injury

Shock treatment is closed-head electrical trauma to the brain. Sufficient electrical current is applied across the patient's skull to produce a grand mal seizure. Usually the individual is shocked three times per week for a total of six or eight times, or more. Sometimes the series will exceed twenty shocks and sometimes patients will be given several series over a period of years. There are patients, usually older women, who have been subjected to a hundred or more shocks.

Originally the patient was simply strapped down to a table, electrodes were applied to the head, and the current was switched on. The electric shock instantly caused unconsciousness and seconds later resulted in a violent grand mal seizure that wracked the body with muscular contractions so strong that bones often were broken.

Since the early 1960s, "modified" electroshock has been the standard practice. The patients are rendered unconscious with an intravenous sedative, and then their muscles are paralyzed with a curare derivative. Because of the paralysis, they cannot breathe, so artificial respiration must be given. The only purpose of this elaborate procedure is to prevent such strong muscular contractions that bones are broken.

The Targets of Shock Treatment

Shock is supposed to be reserved for depression, but doctors will sometimes diagnose depression to justify the treatment. The few surveys available indicate that elderly women are now the most frequently shocked people in the United States.

As I mentioned earlier, shock advocates claim that it is safer than medication in the elderly when in fact it is especially dangerous to them. I believe it's done to elderly women because they are often alone and have no one to defend them from the shock doctors. Also, Medicare covers the treatment, which is highly remunerative and keeps some psychiatric units from going broke.

Research studies show that shock treatment is much too lethal to be unleashed on older patients. In a group of the elderly depressed people subjected to shock, 27 percent died within one year afterward, whereas among a similar group given medications, only 3 percent had died.[6] After two years, 45 percent of the shocked patients had died, but only 9 percent of the nonshock patients were deceased.

The causes of death were varied, including falls and cardiovascular respiratory problems. The increased mortality probably resulted in part from shock-induced memory loss, lethargy, and mental dysfunction that made it impossible for these elderly people to take proper care of themselves.

Meanwhile, the surviving patients were not helped by the shock treatment. Forty-one percent of the shocked patients ended up back in the hospital because of recurring depression, whereas only 15 percent of the nonshock patients were rehospitalized. Overall, twice as many patients relapsed after shock than after more conventional treatments for their depression.

Failing to Tell the Truth

In my clinical and forensic experience, patients and their families are never told the truth about how dangerous shock is; otherwise, they would not consent to it. Shock advocates tend to tell patients that the memory loss is temporary and surrounds the treatment time only, when in reality the memory loss can wipe out years of educational and career knowledge. Women will return home unable to remember their way around their kitchen or what their daughter's wedding was like two years earlier. Nurses, teachers, and other professionals may never again be able to function in their jobs.

Like head injury patients from other causes, such as automobile accidents and lightning strikes, general mental function is often impaired for the rest of their lives. Advocates ignore this by chalking it up to the patient's "mental illness."

A guide to alternative therapies, with a physician as the lead author, said of electric shock treatment, "This technique is almost the exact equivalent of rebooting a computer . . . "[7] Comparing electric shock to rebooting a computer is like comparing a head-on collision to an engine tune-up. More exactly, it's like comparing electrocution to cardiac defibrillation. Neurologist John Friedberg said it in the title to his book, *Electroshock Is Not Good for Your Brain.*

Scientific Evidence for Brain Damage and Dysfunction from Shock

I've written an entire medical book, as well as book chapters and a detailed peer-reviewed scientific report, documenting the harm caused by shock treatment.[8] What follows is an abbreviated summary.

Shock treatment always causes a closed-head injury as manifested by emotional instability, disorientation, confusion, and memory dysfunction. Judgment is so impaired that even shock advocates warn patients and their families that the individual should not make any important decisions for several weeks or more after the treatment. During the treatment, and sometimes for weeks or months afterward, the shock victim becomes either artificially high (euphoria), flattened (apathetic), or both. In medical terms, this is a classic delirium or an organic brain syndrome caused by trauma to the brain.

The question is not "Does shock treatment cause brain dysfunction and damage?" A series of shocks to the head sufficient to cause convulsions will always produce brain dysfunction and damage. The real question is "How completely can a person recover from shock?" From studies of closed-head injury from various causes, we know that recovery is often incomplete. People who suffer from traumatically induced delirium often continue to manifest symptoms for years afterward, sometimes for a lifetime.

Animal studies involving typical clinical doses of shock treatment were conducted in the 1940s and 1950s. They showed brain damage in monkeys, dogs, cats, and rabbits. The damage included bleeding in the brain and neuronal death. After these studies, doctors stopped research on the damaging effects of routine shock in large animals. The doses of electricity were less than those used in modern electroshock. Human autopsy studies showed similar effects to those in shocked animals. After that, doctors stopped doing autopsy studies.

Follow-up studies show that most patients suffer from permanent memory deficits for the life experiences covering months and years prior to the shock treatment. They also have continuing problems with learning and remembering new things.

I have examined patients whose educational and professional experiences were too impaired to permit them to return to work. Some but not all had damage measurable on brain scans.

Long after shock treatment, many patients remain impaired much as if they had been lobotomized. Their personality and emotional life becomes relatively shallow, they are easily irritated, show poor judgment, and lack initiative and self-direction.

It's no surprise that these patients seem lobotomized. They have been subjected to electrical lobotomy. During shock treatment at least one of the electrodes is placed directly over the frontal lobes. It's also no surprise that memory is impaired because the same electrode is also positioned just over the tip of the temporal lobe, an easily traumatized area whose integrity is required for proper memory function. We also know some of the mechanisms by which the damage is caused, including the intensive seizure, extreme hypertension inside the brain, spasms of the blood vessels that cut off oxygenation of the brain and lead to hemorrhages, and electrically induced heat damage and functional disruption.

The seizure itself is also damaging. People who suffer from recurrent spontaneous epileptic seizures often show signs of brain damage. However, electrically induced seizures are much more powerful than ordinary epileptic seizures. When protective measures were not taken during shock, the intensity of the muscular spasms broke bones in the arms, legs, and back, and cracked teeth. Broken bones are almost unheard of during ordinary epileptic seizures.

The Promotional
Campaign for Shock Treatment

Advocates of shock claim that newer methods make it safer. In fact, the methods are neither newer nor safer. I myself administered the supposedly new "modified" ECT more than thirty-five years ago (1963–1964) when I was a psychiatrist in training at Harvard's Massachusetts Mental Health Center. So it's hardly "new." Nor is it safer. Instead, it's more dangerous. The patient is exposed to the additional stress of general anesthesia carried out in a nonsurgical setting in a psychiatric unit. More important, the sedation that's given to the patient makes it more difficult to force the brain to have a seizure. Therefore, modified ECT requires the use of higher amounts of electrical charge than were used in the early animal experiments that showed brain damage and cell death.

ECT for Suicide Prevention

Despite the claims of advocates, there is no evidence that shocking patients reduces their suicidal tendencies. The few studies to address the problem have found no benefit from the shock. In my clinical experience, the brain damage makes people feel more hopeless and resentful, and hence more suicidal. After undergoing shock treatment and before he committed suicide, writer Ernest Hemingway told his biographer that it caused him to lose his memory and his wish to live.

Controlled clinical trials have shown that shock has no positive effect at all or a marginal effect that lasts for only a few weeks. Why a few weeks? That's how long it takes for the worst of the acute brain dysfunction to subside. Until then, the brain is too dysfunctional for the person to feel or to express feelings of depression. At the same time, they can become artificially higher or lapse into apathy.

When I review hospital charts of patients given shock treatment, it's obvious what is happening. If the patient is artificially euphoric from the brain dysfunction, the doctor writes down in the chart "Mood elevated." If the patient becomes apathetic, the doctor writes "No complaints today."

After discharge from the hospital, the patient usually begins a gradual recovery from the worst of the organic brain dysfunction. The depression then returns, now complicated by brain injury. Even advocates of the treatment admit that the effect lasts only a few weeks.

Committing Violence Under
the Influence of Shock Treatment

I was a medical expert in the case of a man who shot a policeman and yet was found not guilty by a jury because the combined effects of shock treatment and drugs had rendered him unable to know right from wrong or to control his impulses. Mr. Clark was undergoing outpatient shock treatment, an especially hazardous way to administer the treatment, but one that is favored by cost-cutting health insurers. He was supposed to be supervised at home round-the-clock, but in fact the hospital did not make sure that this was taking place. Instead, after his second shock treatment he was taken back home and left there to care for his two young children.

When Clark's estranged wife arrived as planned to pick up the children, he was in a state of shock-induced delirium complicated by several psychiatric drugs, including Prozac. He cursed her and refused to give her the children. When a policeman arrived, Clark cursed him as well. Then, as his wife and the policeman sat in a patrol car, Clark came out of his house with two guns blazing from his hips. After an exchange of gunfire, the policeman was slightly wounded and drove off to safety.

Prior to this incident, Clark was a community leader in supporting the police and had recently presented an award to the very policeman he shot. I testified in court that no one recovering from ECT and simultaneously under the influence of multiple psychiatric drugs could be considered competent to control his behavior. The jury agreed with me and he was found not guilty by reason of insanity caused by the effects of electroshock and drugs.

Since Clark had injured a police officer, the jury had to overcome a natural aversion to releasing him. However, they agreed with my testimony concerning the disabling impairment of his brain and mind that was caused by the shock treatment and was worsened by the drugs.

What Should Be Done About Shock Treatment?

Several state legislatures have passed laws banning shock treatment for children. It's now time to ban it for adults as well. Because I favor freedom of choice in medical care, the decision to ban shock was not an easy one for me to make. Ultimately, people are never free to choose shock because the doctors uniformly fail to tell their patients how ineffective and damaging the treatment really is.

Transcranial Stimulation

Transcranial stimulation (TMS) uses magnetic fields to jar the brain into a convulsion. It's another form of shock treatment. Experiments have also been conducted using less intensive stimulation that does not cause convulsions. With this seemingly less traumatic process, studies in animals nonetheless have shown prolonged suppression of brain function.

Although there isn't a vast amount of literature on the potentially harmful effects of these new treatments, I would be wary of becoming an experiment in transcranial electrical stimulation. Remember the basic principle: all drug interventions cause brain malfunction. In regard to physical interventions into the brain, the principle is even more obvious. No one can predict the harm done by tampering with the brain with a method sufficiently potent to affect your mood. A patient might not even be able to tell the difference afterward, because injury to the brain renders individuals less able to evaluate their own mental functioning.

Light Therapy

Some psychiatrists have developed a theory that depression is sometimes caused by seasonal changes in the availability of sunlight. They call it seasonal affective disorder (SAD) and treat patients with high-intensity artificial light for thirty minutes to two hours at a time.

Even among biological psychiatrists, this approach remains controversial. Although it is certainly less harmful than some of the other damaging treatments that doctors impose on depressed patients, it remains fundamentally irrational and misleading.

The coming of winter can make people feel sad for any number of reasons, including a dislike for cold weather or the limitations of indoor activities. But if the seasonal sadness becomes profound or disabling, it's probably caused by a past history of trauma associated with wintertime events, such as the start of school in the fall, anniversaries or birthdays, and Thanksgiving and Christmas holidays. In fact, some people become depressed during the summertime because of their past experiences of abuse or loss during these months of the year.

A patient of mine who was diagnosed with SAD turned out to be harboring guilt feelings about sending a drunken friend out for more beer during a Christmas party several years earlier. The friend died in a collision. The memory was totally forgotten but came up when I did a careful inventory of his fall and wintertime life events.

Your Doctor's Condition

Whether a patient gets shock treatment depends less on the patient's mental condition than on the doctor's mental and moral condition. Many doctors never send people for shock treatment. Some like me would actively intervene if they could to save a patient from shock. Other doctors, by contrast, recommend it for many of their patients. Some doctors, such as Harold Sackeim of the New York State Psychiatric Institute, think that our present shock machines don't deliver nearly enough electrical current to the brain. They want to give two or three times more than required to cause a convulsion.[9] They want to get rid of the safety devices on these machines to amplify the electrical charge delivered to the brain.

Similarly, some hospitals rarely if ever recommend shock. By contrast, a hospital center like Johns Hopkins shocks 10 to20 percent of the patients admitted to its psychiatric wards.[10] That, in my professional opinion, makes Johns Hopkins—and similar medical centers—dangerous places to go for help when you're depressed.

FOURTEEN

The Safety and Efficacy
of Natural Remedies

"Natural products" are not necessarily safer than laboratory-generated chemicals. Some of the most potent psychoactive drugs in the world, including marijuana, alcohol, and the neuroleptic agent Reserpine, are derived from plants. Many toxins are found in plants, including poisonous mushrooms. Having said that, the answer is a qualified "yes"; herbal supplements tend to be safer than FDA-approved antidepressants.

However, it is important to remember the basic rule of brain-disabling treatment: If a drug has an effect on the brain, it is harming the brain. Science has not found or synthesized any psychoactive substances that improve normal brain function. Instead, all of them impair brain function. To a great extent, it's a matter of dosage. Herbs are usually recommended in doses that fall short of producing serious adverse effects or intoxication. But antidepressants are typically prescribed in doses that cause a wide variety of adverse effects in most patients and significantly harm a great many people.

The Usefulness of Some
"Alternative" Treatments

Saw palmetto, for example, is an excellent treatment for benign prostatic hypertrophy. Although drugs and herbs are too freely taken by most people, the use of these substances is much more rational in medicine than in psychiatry and psychology. In medicine, the problem usually originates in the body, and it certainly affects the body. Judicious physical interventions into the physical body can make sense. But in psychiatry, none of the problems are proven to originate in the brain. Furthermore, the brain is far more intricate and vulnerable than any other organ of the body. Tampering with it can produce profound psychological and mental dysfunctions.

St. John's Wort

St. John's wort is by far the most commonly suggested alternative herbal treatment for depression. It is derived from *Hypericum perforatum,* a flowering plant that grows wild throughout much of the world. *Wort* is the Old English term for plant. According to Gale Maleskey (1999) in *Nature's Medicines,* "The name St. John's wort may have come about because red or bloodlike spots appear on hypericum leaves in June, around the anniversary of the beheading of St. John the Baptist. During the Middle Ages, on the saint's anniversary, peasants slept with cuttings of the plant under their pillows. They hoped that St. John would appear in their dreams, bless them, and give them life for another year."

Although the mystical use of St. John's wort may seem ridiculous to us now, I'm not sure there's more rational justification for using it to cure an essentially psychological and spiritual state, depression. Nonetheless, in Germany, St. John's wort is a government-approved medication for depression. In the United States, unlike Germany, it has not received official government sanction, but it is more commonly used than the FDA-approved antidepressants.

Although *Hypericum* is often considered the most active substance, St. John's wort is a mixture of many different potentially psychoactive substances, and it's unclear which of them have the most significant effects. Some of its components may inhibit the removal of serotonin from the synapse in a similar fashion to the SSRIs. But a range of chemicals will be affecting your brain and mind if you take this herb.

Scientific Studies of St. John's Wort

Clinical trials have shown that St. John's wort has some beneficial effect on depression, but remember that clinical trials are almost always conducted by advocates and are often manipulated to produce the desired outcome. Clinical studies also show a relatively safe profile of adverse effects. For people who feel that they must try a psychoactive substance for its potential antidepressant effects, St. John's wort may be a better bet than any of the regularly prescribed FDA-approved antidepressants.

Almost all the herbal textbooks I've looked at have warned not to rely on St. John's wort for treating severe depression or suicidal tendencies. They recommend instead that people rely on prescription antidepressants. This is pure psychopharmaceutical propaganda. When Prozac was tested on hospitalized patients for FDA approval, it was not effective either. Suicidal patients are excluded from most antidepressant studies. If anything, as I've already indicated, antidepressants worsen severe depression and suicidal tendencies.

It's dangerous to rely on any chemical substance, including St. John's wort or prescription antidepressants, if you're feeling suicidal. If you feel in danger of harming yourself, a caring, experienced psychotherapist is a far better resource than a drug. People rarely commit suicide when they have good rapport with a therapist to whom they can turn, especially a therapist who is willing to involve other people in your life who care about you.

Adverse Effects of St. John's Wort

No psychoactive agent is harmless. In particular, there are significant dangers·surrounding potential drug interactions. St. John's wort should not be combined with other antidepressants. Toxic reactions may develop because of overstimulation of serotonin. Since Prozac can remain in the body for many weeks after the last dose, St. John's wort should not be taken for three weeks to a month after stopping Prozac. Taking St. John's wort with monoamine oxidase inhibitors, a particular hazardous class of antidepressants, is especially likely to cause toxic reactions.

St. John's wort may also interfere with the effectiveness of a number of other drugs by speeding up the activity of a liver enzyme, cytochrome P450. As a result, the liver will destroy these substances more rapidly, diminishing their effectiveness. Anyone planning to take St. John's wort along with other medications should check with a physician and with some of the books listed in the endnotes to this chapter.[1]

Once again, it should be apparent that most psychoactive substances have the potential to cause serious problems.

Other Remedies

Because depression responds so well to placebo, false claims for effectiveness are made for many different substances. Natural remedies for depression are discussed in a variety of books that are readily available in libraries and bookstores.[2] However, none of the herbs or supplements have been researched anywhere near as thoroughly or used as widely as St. John's wort, and some of them are much more dangerous.

Taking herbs and supplements may seem to help some people, but it's basically a flawed and misleading approach. Unless you are suffering from a genuine physical disorder, such as hypothyroidism, there's little likelihood that your feelings of depression arise from a physical disorder. If your depression is the result of a physical disorder, you should diagnose and treat the physical disorder itself without complicating your physical and mental condition by taking antidepressants. Chapter 11 surveys the kinds of physical problems that can cause or contribute to depression.

Devoting time and energy to finding the "right" natural remedy can easily detour you from dealing with the personal and psychological issues in your life. If you find yourself relying heavily on these substances to heal emotional suffering or discomfort, you probably need to redirect your efforts to understanding and overcoming the more painful aspects of your life.

FIFTEEN

How Drug Companies Can Deceive the Courts, the Medical Profession, and the Public

In the early 1990s, I was asked to be the medical consultant to several dozen "combined Prozac suits." Most of the suits charged Eli Lilly and Co. with fraud in covering up Prozac's tendency to cause suicide and violence. An Indiana court had combined the suits for the purpose of conducting a single discovery process. One attorney was put in charge of collecting the drug company's records, sifting through and analyzing them, and developing the basic approach to bringing the lawsuits.

I was hired as the medical consultant to the combined Prozac cases by the first attorney put in charge of them. When Leonard Ring, a highly regarded Chicago attorney, replaced him, Ring continued to work with me as his medical expert. Unfortunately, Ring died and was replaced by Paul Smith, a Dallas attorney. Smith became the leader of the entire legal assault on Eli Lilly and Co. and prepared to bring the first case to court.

Unlike every other attorney who has ever hired me, Smith spent almost no time going over the case with me. I was left on my own to evaluate enormous amounts of material and to develop the substance of my future testimony.

The first Prozac case to come to court revolved around Joseph Wesbecker, a Louisville, Kentucky, man who perpetrated a murderous onslaught at his former place of work. The case was complicated because Wesbecker had displayed serious emotional problems and overt hostility toward his former employers before he ever took Prozac. In 1989, although he was doing relatively well, psychiatrist Lee Coleman of Kentucky[1] added Prozac to his treatment regimen. On the routine follow-up visit a month later, the doctor found that Wesbecker had become delusional. The doctor wrote, "Patient seems to have deteriorated." Wesbecker was "weeping" and displayed an "increased level of agitation and anger." In the record, Coleman questioned whether Prozac might be causing the patient's worsening condition and he stopped the medication.

Three days later, with most of the Prozac still active in his body, Wesbecker took an arsenal to his former place of work, shot twenty people, killed eight, and then killed himself. Eli Lilly and Co. was sued by a large number of victims of the shootings and their surviving families.

In my analysis of the case, I concluded that Wesbecker already harbored anger toward his former employers, but that Prozac had made him so agitated, paranoid, and psychotic that he could no longer control his existing aggressive impulses. I also concluded that Wesbecker's doctor should not be accused of malpractice, because Eli Lilly and Co. had withheld the information that could have warned him not to prescribe Prozac to a man who was already struggling with violent impulses. At the time, Coleman had no way of knowing, for example, that Prozac commonly caused akathisia, a disorder that can drive an already depressed patient into a dangerous state of *agitated* depression. He had no way of knowing that Eli Lilly and Co. possessed data confirming very high rates of agitation and increased rates of suicide attempts on Prozac. He had no way of knowing that Prozac caused psychotic mania in patients who had never before undergone mania. Eli Lilly and Co. had hidden all this data from the public and the profession, and some of it from the FDA as well.[2]

My refusal to support a malpractice suit against Coleman may have alerted Smith to the fact that I could not be manipulated into saying anything he wanted me to say in court. From then on, I remained his main medical expert in the Wesbecker case against the drug company, but for reasons not yet apparent to me, Smith had little or nothing to do with me.

Caught in the Middle of a Fix

When I arrived in Louisville, Kentucky, for the trial, I was shocked to find out that Paul Smith had sequestered me in a hotel that was miles away from where he and the other attorneys were staying. In other cases, attorneys have put me in the same hotel with them to make it easier to review facts and issues together. When I telephoned my wife, Ginger, and told her what was going on, she became suspicious. But neither of us could guess what might be happening behind my back.

My suspicions turned into grave concerns when Smith refused to discuss my upcoming testimony with me. He wanted me to get on the stand and respond to whatever he happened to ask me. Attorneys in huge suits like this usually spend many hours and even days going over the testimony in advance with the expert. I was now both suspicious and frightened about what lay ahead of me.

Withholding Evidence from Their Own Expert

In the few days remaining before I went on the stand, I spent hours alone in Smith's temporary office in a Louisville law firm while he conducted the ongoing trial. I now found out that he had kept many relevant documents from me, including a detailed, color-coded chart about Joseph Wesbecker's childhood that had been created by the drug company from its investigations.

When I asked for a copy of the biographical chart, Smith refused, and only gave in after I vigorously demanded it. Smith also continued to refuse to discuss my testimony with me, so I wrote out my testimony for him in the form of dozens of note cards with prepared questions for him to ask me. After another confrontation, he agreed to ask me some of my proposed questions on the stand.

Increasingly I felt like I was being set up, but why or to what end?

The Testimony

My testimony went well despite Paul Smith's obstructionist tactics. Much of Eli Lilly's cross-examination of me was based on the childhood chart that Smith had unsuccessfully tried to keep from me, but fortunately I had it in front of me on the witness stand. In retrospect, I was obviously being set up to look foolish and make Eli Lilly and Co. look good. But it went awry because I found the sequestered chart and could answer the questions in minute detail.

With some exceptions, Smith asked me most of the questions I had written out for him on my note cards. He probably feared that I would figure out the scheme if he refused to ask me any of the pertinent questions that I'd worked so hard to present him.

Nonetheless, attorney Smith did refuse to ask me on the stand about some of the most important discoveries I had made, many of which are described throughout this book. For example, I found the material described in Chapter 6 about the Prozac label originally listing "depression" as a commonly reported adverse reaction to Prozac. I brought him a copy of the label charges showing how it had been scratched out at the last minute, but he refused to let me use this striking new evidence that the company knew that its drug could cause depression and yet allowed the fact to be removed from the label.

The Jury Verdict

The jury came back in favor of the drug company by a divided 9–3 vote. One more vote against Eli Lilly and Co. would have hung the jury and created a public relations nightmare for Prozac.

However, soon after the trial, presiding judge John W. Potter concluded that Eli Lilly and Co. had fixed the trial. The drug company had secretly given a huge sum of money to Smith and his clients in return for which Smith had presented a watered-down case to the jury.[3] No wonder Smith tried to stifle my testimony. In return for a mammoth advance settlement, he had agreed to present a weakened case in court, and I was ruining the scheme.

The judge, meanwhile, was especially outraged because toward the trial's conclusion he had asked both sides if they had made a secret settlement, and both sides had denied it.[4] Smith and Eli Lilly and Co. then went on with the rigged trial to make it come out right for the drug company.

In retrospect, it's also obvious that the aim of discrediting me as an expert witness for future Prozac suits was also a part of the overall settlement. The strategy failed only because I had prepared my testimony despite Smith and because I had found critical documents he had purposely withheld from me.

In keeping with Smith's determination both to lose the trial and to discredit me as the key expert, he allowed Eli Lilly and Co. to attack me during their summation to the jury without making any attempt to rebut their criticism in his own summation. He could have reminded the jury, for example, that the drug company had failed to cross-examine me about any of my scientific observations on such things as their secret study showing that Prozac increases the suicide rate in depressed patients.

The Final Outcome

Judge Potter decided to change the verdict of the trial. He threw out the jury verdict and changed it to a settlement with prejudice by Eli Lilly and Co. Both Paul Smith and Eli Lilly and Co. then appealed the judge's decision to the Kentucky Supreme Court. The supreme court concluded that the drug company had "manipulated" the judicial system and further opined that Eli Lilly and Co. might even have committed "fraud."

After Judge Potter changed the verdict, he prepared to disclose the seemingly enormous amount of money that had been paid (I would estimate hundreds of millions of dollars). At this moment, Eli Lilly and Co. forced Judge Potter to withdraw himself from the proceedings. The new judge concluded that the amounts paid by Eli Lilly and Co. were so large that their disclosure would harm the drug company. The case ended with the invalidation of the jury verdict and with the open admission that the Wesbecker trial had been rigged. But there was no disclosure about the amounts of money that changed hands.

Paul Smith, in the process, settled all his cases with Eli Lilly and Co. and retired. Smith once told me that the case had put him a million dollars in debt, but at its conclusion he was wealthy enough to retire.

Smith refused to cooperate with the other attorneys in the combined suits. His research and discovery documents were seemingly lost, greatly hampering future suits.

Although the mass media had covered the original fake victory by Eli Lilly and Co, only the British news agency, Reuters, made any mention of the reversal against the drug company. As a result of the media silence, the faked trial was a massive legal, public relations, and political victory for Eli Lilly and Co.

My Own Reactions

I was extraordinarily disillusioned by the fixing of the Wesbecker trial but managed eventually to recover and to continue to act as a medical expert in increasing numbers of legal cases, including numerous ones against Prozac and Eli Lilly and Co. All of my cases against the drug company have been settled without going to court.

The Growing Impact of Drug Companies

The Wesbecker trial indicates the degree to which a powerful drug company can and will influence American society, including the courts and the media. This influence reaches into the very heart of organized psychiatry and medicine.

As a life member of my profession's most influential professional organization, the American Psychiatric Association (APA), I am appalled at how it is dominated by the drug companies. The American Psychiatric Association was going broke in the early 1970s until its leadership consciously decided to go into partnership with the drug companies. As I documented in *Toxic Psychiatry*, I traced the decisionmaking process in the minutes of the association's board of directors.

Although my use of the word "partnership" may seem unnecessarily strong, it's actually their own word for the relationship between drug companies and the psychiatric association. In a letter published in the *New York Times,* I criticized the American Psychiatric Association for accepting a "donation" of $1 million cash from the Upjohn Corporation, which makes Xanax and Halcion. In response to my letter, the medical director of the American Psychiatric Association wrote that his organization has a "partnership" with the drug companies.[5]

It's a very profitable partnership. The drug companies pour millions into the association's coffers through direct contributions and through support of specific activities such as the APA's staff, journals, conferences, and promotional activities. The association has always refused to disclose the overall amount, but in a surprising recent admission, the president of the American Psychiatric Association, Daniel Borenstein, lamented that "Approximately one-third of APA's annual income is derived from the pharmaceutical industry."

Of course, many leading experts on psychiatric drugs have close ties with the American Psychiatric Association and this in turn gives them another strong association with the drug companies.

Basically, it's one powerful interest group—what I have labeled the Psychopharmaceutical Complex.

The HMOs (Health Maintenance Organizations), PPOs (Preferred Provider Organizations), and other health insurers also support the use of drugs rather than psychotherapy and other human services. They want to cut the cost of mental health services and favor doctors who are willing to substitute "Med Checks"—ten- to fifteen-minute prescription review sessions—for more lengthy psychotherapy or family therapy sessions. The HMOs limit psychiatric benefits and encourage physicians to prescribe psychiatric medications and to see their patients as infrequently as possible. The PPOs choose psychiatrists and other physicians for their networks on the basis of their willingness to do the same. Increasingly, independent psychiatrists and psychotherapists have to go through hoops to justify any amount of psychotherapy for their patients.

You can have endless visits to the doctor for drug prescriptions, but any visits for psychotherapy are likely to be challenged or minimally funded. I know therapists who have quit their private practices rather than continue to hassle with the insurance companies about not referring their patients for medication.

The Role of the Federal Government

Most people realize that Washington increasingly dances to the tune of corporate America, but they don't realize to what extent federal agencies push psychiatric drugs for the benefit of the pharmaceutical industry. The National Institute of Mental Health (NIMH) has transformed itself into an aggressive extension of the pharmaceutical industry. On their behalf, NIMH conducts expensive, highly biased clinical trials. Most shamefully, NIMH is currently planning to conduct studies of stimulant drugs on four- to six-year-old children diagnosed with ADHD. NIMH organizes so-called educational campaigns like "Depression Awareness Week" that promote drugs. It regularly issues comments and even press releases touting biological psychiatry and drugs.

The influence of the drug companies on federal agencies cannot be exaggerated. In the midst of the controversy over Prozac causing suicide and violence, Steven Paul, director of research at NIMH, was hired away to become vice president of Eli Lilly and Co. During the transition, he defended Prozac at a critical time of controversy about the drug's capacity to cause suicide and violence.

The Food and Drug Administration (FDA) has forsaken its watchdog role. Instead, FDA officials climb like puppies into the laps of drug company executives who might some day hire them at enormous salaries. Paul Leber was for many years the director of the FDA's psychiatric drug section; now he makes a living as a consultant to drug companies.

Even the U.S. Department of Education has taken on the role of drug pusher by promoting stimulants like Ritalin for schoolchildren. The agency finds it easier to subdue children with drugs than to promote more imaginative educational reform and better teaching.

The drug industry, the insurance business, professional organizations like the American Psychiatric Association, drug company funded parent groups like NAMI and CHADD, and the government constitute the Psychopharmaceutical Complex. To learn more of the details, you can read chapters on the Psychopharmaceutical Complex in several of my other books, beginning with *Toxic Psychiatry* (1991) and most recently in *Talking Back to Ritalin*. My main point is that physicians and patients alike cannot trust the information that they routinely receive about drugs, including SSRI antidepressants.

Whoever controls the flow of information controls the kinds of choice you and I can make. Nowadays, the flow of information about critical health care issues is even more controlled than the delivery of health care itself. Put simply, important facts about psychiatric drugs are withheld from the public and even from the doctors, making informed choices nearly impossible.

SIXTEEN

How to Overcome Depression: Suggestions for Patients and Therapists Alike

What is the solution to depression? The answer is straightforward but difficult to implement: Find the inspiration to love life and then make choices that are consistent with your ethics and your happiness.

Depression is an emotional statement that life matters and has meaning, and that we are deeply distressed by how it's been going. Depressed feelings are signals that we need to replace old self-defeating ways of thinking and acting with new approaches based on treasuring our own life and the lives of those whom we touch. However, the path toward overcoming depression can be confusing, difficult, and treacherous. You may be frustrated in your marriage because your husband or wife doesn't cherish you. But you are stifled in regard to taking action because you have learned in childhood that "men can't change" or "women just want to use you." Or you may be inhibited in acting because of childhood beliefs that "no one could love me anyway." Or you may think, "I've never seen a happy marriage, so there's no point to leaving or to trying to improve this marriage or to hope for a better one."

Or you may be frustrated in regard to your work life. You want to seek a new job but believe that there are no interesting jobs, that no one would want you, that you couldn't possibly make money doing something worthwhile, or that you don't deserve to be well paid for doing something that you love.

A principled guide, such as a therapist or counselor, can often help us to discover our personal blocks to the pursuit of happiness, and help us to formulate principles of living that are ethical, productive, and at times joyful.

Meanwhile, the ways of finding renewed motivation and inspiration to love life are as varied as life itself. People have learned to overcome depression and to create a principled, loving life through books and contemplation, through romantic love and family life, through nature, through creative work, through exercise, through the healing passage of time, and ultimately through the courage and determination to change their lives for the better. The process can involve an infinite variety of psychological, moral, spiritual, and religious practices.

By ethical and moral practices, I mean those that involve respect for the rights of others. By spiritual practices, I mean those that focus on love and the pursuit of higher ideals whether or not they include formal religion or a concept of God.

The Moral Context of Therapy

People become vulnerable to feelings of depression when all the alternatives seem unfairly bleak or because guilt, shame, and anxiety inhibit them from making an otherwise positive choice. Depressed people usually have a dim awareness of a potentially better life but no longer believe it's possible for them. They have lapsed into that particular form of helplessness and hopelessness called depression.

Depressed persons feel paralyzed in their ability to make satisfying or meaningful choices. They fear that there are no viable alternatives, no choices that will make any real difference, and that ultimately they must in some way bear the blame for their fate. Thus, depression can often be understood as based on moral conflicts from which the individual can imagine no escape.

It's rare for people to come to therapy with an awareness of the moral nature of their problem. Yet it will readily come to light when the therapist asks why the problems cannot be resolved by one or another choice or action. At that point the individual is likely to declare that the alternatives are "bad," "idealistic" "wrong," or otherwise unacceptable or unrealistic.

The thwarting of important personal needs or aspirations commonly leads to depressed feelings. The underlying cause often revolves around conflicts between values or between moral codes and personal desires. For example, a woman may wish to leave her abusive husband but find it morally incompatible with her religious upbringing. Or a man may want to leave his wife but finds it incompatible with his wish to be a good father to the children he will leave behind.

There are, of course, no easy solutions to many of the conflicts that arise in life. The therapist must be prepared to keep an open mind about the patient's moral values. At times the therapist should disclose his own values when they tend to conflict with the patient's. Only a fully informed patient can decide if the therapist's values are getting in the way of finding his or her own solutions.

Drugs Versus Therapy and Life

Tragically, the mental health professions and their interest groups have convinced many people that there are only two alternatives for dealing with seriously depressed feelings: drugs or electroshock. Nowadays it can seem radical to suggest psychotherapy as an alternative. In reality, people commonly overcome depressed feelings, even the most severe kind, by an infinite number of approaches that inspire and motivate them to take a fresh, more engaged approach to life. Often other people play a role in providing encouragement and guidance, including family, friends, therapists, religious counselors, and authors. Sometimes people make the change without turning for help to anyone else, but that is by far the hardest and most hazardous way.

Because I am a psychiatrist and a psychotherapist, I will devote this concluding chapter to psychological therapy as a method of overcoming depressed feelings. But I want the reader to remember that psychotherapy is but one approach, and that among psychotherapies, there are many different schools and different personal approaches.

Psychotherapy for Depression

Therapeutic processes are extremely varied and often overlap with ethical and spiritual approaches. One therapeutic approach, called cognitive therapy, focuses on how we think. It emphasizes replacing self-defeating ideas or concepts with more positive and effective ones. Behavioral therapies, by contrast, focus on changing how we act. Insight therapies often aim at uncovering painful early childhood experiences and more recent stressors that have contributed to feelings of depression. Insight therapies also try to examine how the individual's reactions continue to impede progress. Interpersonal therapies emphasize a positive relationship with the therapist. Choice therapy urges the individual to embrace his or her capacity to make decisions. Existential therapy concerns itself with the individual's need to choose meaningful values for guiding one's life.

Biblical therapy draws on lessons from the Bible and tends to emphasize moral exhortation. Spiritual counseling is a broader term that describes a variety of approaches that attempt to be consistent with higher ideals, a belief in God, or more specific theological concerns.

Humanistic therapy is perhaps the most encompassing term. It includes empowering individuals by bringing out their inherent capacities to choose, to behave ethically, and to love. Humanistic therapy, unlike the philosophy of humanism, by no means excludes a belief in religion or God.

By now it should be apparent that it is mistaken to speak of "therapy" as if it were a monolithic approach to helping people. Not only the theoretical models but also the practices of individual therapists can vary enormously. The therapist's particular personality, for example, plays a major role in any therapy. Therapy involves people helping people, and nothing matters as much as the ethics, values, wisdom and determination of the particular people involved in the enterprise.

Many if not most therapists use a combination of approaches, depending on their own personal preference and on the needs or desires of the patient. My approach varies somewhat from patient to patient but overall I try to create a safe and caring relationship in which to explore the nature of the patient's suffering and conflict, and through which to help the patient find more effective approaches to life. Although my writing has emphasized the role of empathy and love in therapy, I have avoided the temptation to try to create a new approach with a new name and instead draw on the best of the various schools.

I also try to be "real" with my clients so that they get to know me much in the way my friends know me. The main difference is that I do not talk at length about myself and instead focus almost exclusively on them.

I believe that good therapy helps the patient learn how to heal and especially how to share love and understanding with others in their lives. It also encourages patients to learn how to protect themselves during conflict and how to remain independent within loving relationships. Therapy that involves couples and families is often the most effective because it teaches people to care for and to heal each other, yet maintain their independence.

What to Expect from the Therapy Relationship

As a patient or client, you are hiring a professional to help to you to improve your life. Keep in mind that you are paying the bill and that you should receive a good, even a wonderful service in return. Despite the professional aspect—the fee, the focus on getting help, the limits on intimacy, the restraints on contacts outside the office—therapy remains a human relationship. Much as finding a friend or lifetime partner, you may need to try several therapists and to change therapists along the way before finding one that inspires you to live a better, happier life.

Some people think of therapy as "artificial" and "like buying friendship." To some extent this is true, but that's not necessarily negative. When we pay for therapy, we should expect to purchase an ideal relationship, one in which we can feel cared for and understood without the dangers inherent in less structured nonprofessional relationships.

In our daily relationships, caring and empathy should of course be mutual. The same is true in therapy. If a mutually caring relationship does not develop, you won't gain the maximum benefit and you may even end up feeling injured by the repetition of yet another emotionally handicapped relationship in which you neither give nor receive enough mutual respect and caring.

People, intentionally or not, are the major cause of suffering in people. Similarly, people, intentionally or not, are the greatest source of healing for people. In therapy we are given the opportunity to explore and even to reexperience our relationships with people, and to heal ourselves in the context of a caring professional relationship.

The Effect of Depressing Personal Relationships

Because of my public profile, I've been chosen as a "doctor of last resort" by many patients. Although I discourage people from imagining that I have the ability to rescue them or that I'm the only person who could help them, I have learned a lot from my experience in seeing patients who have done poorly in previous psychiatric treatment.

People usually remain trapped in depressed feelings because they have not been able to escape from depressing relationships in their lives. Sometimes these emotionally enslaving relationships are with people from the past who may no longer be alive. Often they are with people with whom they continue to live.

When a new patient of mine says that he or she hasn't been able to get over feeling depressed for years, I begin in the first session to inquire about the nature of their relationships with their parents, their spouse and children, their friends, and their previous psychiatrists or therapists. Very commonly, the persistently depressed person is compulsively trying to placate an oppressive and often depressed parent. Even if the contacts with the parent take place only once every few weeks by telephone or e-mail, they may be enough to reinforce the person's feelings of worthlessness and guilt.

Unfortunately, it can be very hard for victimized people to grasp how much their relationships contribute to their suffering. They often feel guilty about evaluating a parent's effect on them. However, the patient's husband or wife is likely to report that every phone call from the parents ends with the patient feeling depressed and withdrawn.

A depressing relationship with a husband or wife can also keep a person mired down in a lifetime of self-hate and despair. Many people feel trapped in marriages or long-term relationships that make both participants feel guilty and worthless. Out of fear of losing each other, they end up interfering with each other's attempts to build a more independent, creative life.

Why don't they stand up for themselves or leave the relationship? Underneath it all, they may still love each other. Or they may have a moral or religious commitment to staying married. Or they may feel dreadfully frightened and guilty at the thought of questioning the marriage or relationship.

The Effect of Depressing Therapy Relationships

Relationships with oppressive, depressing therapists—especially psychiatrists—are a very common cause for people failing to overcome their persistent feelings of depression. Working with a therapist who lacks enthusiasm for life and who views you as suffering from a "disorder" can in itself become very depressing.

Nowadays, many if not most doctors and therapists have very negative ideas about depressed people, including that they suffer from biochemical imbalances and genetic defects and that they need to take drugs for the rest of their lives. As a result, individual patients can find themselves going from one depressing doctor to another. Having failed in their efforts to get help, these patients actually end up believing the negative view of depression held by their doctors.

Even a seemingly vital and caring doctor can nowadays end up prescribing antidepressant drugs. The drugs are given out so freely that anyone who's been depressed for a while is probably taking several different drugs at once. Nothing reinforces depression more than having your brain befuddled by psychiatric drugs, unless it has having your mind befuddled by false ideas about the biological or genetic origin of your suffering.

At best, antidepressants can only mute the signals of depression or substitute an artificial sense of well-being. Either way, the underlying personal conflicts will not be identified, addressed, and resolved. Instead, the individual will tend to remain mired down in the same depressing viewpoints and situations. Thus, antidepressants encourage us to continue submitting to frustrating, unsatisfying ways of looking at and living life. In the process, they end up impairing our very ability to think and feel. By limiting our ability to experience or to express our thoughts, feelings, and willpower, they *force* us to remain mired down in a tragically limited rendition of what our lives could be.

Since depression is a particular way of thinking and feeling in response to disappointment and loss, the best solution requires learning to overcome these negative thoughts and feelings. It stands to reason that misguided, self-defeating ideas can only be changed through embracing better ideas. We don't give people drugs to change them from one religion or another or from one political ideology to another. We may hope that life will teach the person a better viewpoint and, if we have the opportunity, we may try to change the person's viewpoint through rational discussion. But we know we are dealing with thoughts and feelings that need to be influenced by experience and communication.

Similarly, if you have the depressing idea that your life offers no worthwhile alternatives, you need a change in attitude, not a mind-altering drug. Or if you have feelings such as hopelessness or despair that are undermining your life, you need to find encouragement and hope. You don't need to have your feelings artificially blunted or elevated. You need to find new ways of thinking and feeling about your life, and ultimately, you need a new approach to making choices that are more ethically consistent and fulfilling.

Identifying Depressing Relationships

If you've been depressed for years without getting any better, ask yourself the following kinds of questions:

"Am I in contact with a parent who is depressed and depressing." Conversely, *"Do my contacts with my parent make me feel cherished and treasured?"* Many people remain locked into relationships with parents who undermine them on the phone, by letter and e-mail, and in person. Ask your wife or husband, or check for yourself, to see how you feel after a phone call with your mother or father. Ask yourself how you feel when it's time to visit them at Thanksgiving or Christmas. When we do not feel cherished and loved by people who are supposed to love us, we often react by feeling depressed.

"Am I in a marriage or intimate friendship that too often leaves me feeling unloved or to blame for all the failures in the relationship? Am I, for some reason, feeling unable to improve or to leave the relationship?" Conversely, ask yourself, *"Do I feel cherished and treasured by my spouse?"* Many people think that marriage

is supposed to bottom out over the years at a relatively bland emotional level. In reality, a good marriage continues to mature in new and wonderful directions. People continue to want to be loved, and in the absence of that love, they can easily become depressed.

"Has my self-esteem and confidence been undermined by being told that I have a clinical depression or a biochemical imbalance? Whenever I had a painful or frightening feelings, did my doctor tinker with my drugs instead of encouraging me to explore and to understand the feelings? Have I been prescribed a series of psychiatric medications, all of which have failed in the long run to help me? Ultimately, does my doctor seem brimming over with enthusiasm for life and for me, or does he or she seem depressed?" Conversely, ask yourself, "Have I been treated as a human being who can understand his or her life, and make better choices for the future? Have I felt valued and understood by my psychiatrist or therapist? Did we have a really good relationship in which I felt understood and cared for? Have the sessions empowered me to believe in my own psychological strength and my own ability to make positive choices for myself?"

Helping Very Depressed People

The more depressed people become, the more important it is for the therapist to create a hopeful, encouraging, caring relationship. In other words, the sadder the patient has become, the more important it is for the therapist to be a joyful, optimistic person. There's no way to fake enthusiasm or confidence; therefore, therapists cannot be fully effective until they feel good about themselves and their own lives.

In my work, the quality of my professional relationship with my patient remains central to everything I do. As my patients talk about their lives, I try to develop an empathic relationship in which they can feel that their suffering is understood. An empathic relationship helps to dispel the loneliness and isolation that the depressed and anxious person almost always experiences. A good relationship inspires confidence in the therapist and in the patients' own ability to find solutions.

At the same time, I try to instill confidence that the problems can be resolved through identifying previously self-defeating ways of relating and by developing new and better approaches to family life, friendship, work, and creativity.

In the early stages of the therapy relationship, I'm always aware of my own attitudes and viewpoints and how I can bring the best that I have to the situation. Some people need and want me to be more formal, others want me to be more casual and relaxed, some people want me to talk a lot, and others want me to listen a lot. Some people feel the need to learn a little about me as a person and as a professional, whereas others find that distracting. Some people are always serious, and other people want a little levity. Some people enjoy my getting them a cup of tea or a glass of water; others don't want to disrupt the work. Some people want to read my books, others have no desire to do so. Many people like to be greeted by my newest "therapy assistant," my Shetland sheep dog, Maggie; other people understandably feel that dogs are distracting in a session. As a patient, you have the right to expect your therapist to do his or her best to make you feel comfortable and to converse in a fashion that seems productive to you.

Of course, there are limits to any therapist's flexibility and versatility, and that's one of the reasons that patients should shop carefully before deciding on a therapist. But in an empathic, caring relationship, it's often possible to make adjustments that increase the comfort and security of the other person. This is true in every kind of human relationship.

Welcoming the Depressed Feelings

Doctors can become frightened or even overwhelmed by a patient's depressed feelings, and that can lead them to take drastic harmful actions, such as prescribing psychoactive drugs or shock treatment. Therapists need to know how to welcome their patient's feelings of depression. After all, these are the feelings that drove the patient to seek help, so it's an advantage to have the suffering come out fully in the session.

These depressed feelings are signals of underlying frustration and despair, and can provide a window in the sources of the problem. At the height of a depressed feeling, an individual can be guided to find and to express the core of despair—the conflict and torment that has been buried within the gloom and hopelessness.

Extremely negative feelings of almost any kind have this positive aspect of signaling the underlying needs and frustrations of a potentially powerful but thwarted human being. Always remember that unless people deeply cared about their lives, they wouldn't become so wretchedly disappointed and discouraged. In this vein, I tell my patients, "You wouldn't be so horribly depressed if you didn't have a sense of how good life can be. You're not indifferent toward your life—you hate it. That means you want something better—much, much better. I want to help you create a life that you can love." I say this somewhat differently with each of my patients but basically I'm communicating that the intensity of their suffering signals the intensity of their life force, and that I'm glad to be working with someone who feels such passion about life.

Since patients feel frightened and even guilty about their depressed feelings, they can experience enormous relief when the therapist welcomes the feelings and wants to remain open to their suffering. When a psychiatrist instead offers a drug, he or she in effect says, "I can't bear your feelings either; let me help you rid yourself of them." The prescription of drugs can easily become a statement by the doctor that "You and I cannot do anything about your feelings, so let's make you feel numb instead."

The only way to understand feelings is to eagerly invite them to come out in the open. Once their source is understood, the individual can use them to motivate and to guide change for the better. Feelings of depression that used to be treated as intolerable can become welcome signals that the individual needs to become aware of a source of stress or disappointment. In this way, depression can function as a motivation and a guide for discovering that something harmful has happened or is taking place. The individual can say, in effect, "Now I know what's making me so miserable. I've fallen into the trap of succumbing to my spouse's anger, or I've again forgotten to take care of my own needs for love, or once again I'm working much too hard." The depressed feelings not only point toward the problem, they can motivate the individual to find the courage to change his or her life for the better.

Dealing with Emotional Emergencies

As a helping person, the single most important thing in dealing with emotional emergencies is to avoid having one yourself. When distraught patients realize that their "emergency" doesn't strike a similar panic or dread in their therapist, their crisis is likely to begin resolving on the spot. "After all," the patient tends to conclude, "If my therapist isn't freaked out about my wanting to die, maybe I can handle it too."

Therefore, the more my patients feel that they are desperate, the harder I try to calm myself down. When I remain calm, my patients are likely to calm down as well. They will feel that I've got the situation under control, so they can relax. Eventually they realize that they themselves can take control.

Doctors commonly make the mistake of adopting the same viewpoint as the patient. When the distraught patient feels like the world is coming to an end or that suicide is the only alternative, doctors too often tend to confirm the fears by raising the drug dose, recommending hospitalization, or even inflicting electroshock on the patient. By accepting the patient's fear the doctor actually contributes to wrecking the patient's life and world.

In the doctor's office or in the emergency room, a confident doctor who is able to relate in an empathic fashion should be able to handle almost any emotional "emergency" without resort to drugs or restraints. In all of my thirty-plus years of full-time psychiatric practice, I've never started a patient on psychiatric drugs, and I haven't recommended hospitalization on more than a dozen occasions in all those years. Furthermore, as I mentioned in Chapter 9, I have never involuntarily hospitalized anyone during my entire career since entering private practice in 1968.

Because I don't use any of these "emergency" techniques, I have to work very hard to communicate with my patients and to help them find immediate, if partial, solutions to their most acute problems. As a result of not drugging people and not forcing them into hospitals, I have to try very hard to remain empathic and understanding toward my patients and to be very available to them in times of need. In seemingly desperate situations, I try to involve the patient's family, friends, and anyone else who cares about the individual. But I don't resort to force and I don't start the patient on drugs.

Expressing My Views
on Drugs to Patients

Consistent with my respect for the autonomy of my patients, I don't discourage them from seeking medication from other doctors. In fact, since medication is so freely available, I'm not depriving them of freedom of choice by refusing to start them on medication myself. As a result, my patients occasionally seek an antidepressant from another doctor during treatment with me. It probably happens less than once a year and usually these patients decide that the drug is interfering with their recovery.

If patients are already taking psychiatric drugs when they come to see me, I don't push them to stop taking them unless a dangerous drug reaction becomes apparent. I will discuss my views and offer them my books to read, such as *Your Drug May Be Your Problem: How and Why to Stop Taking Psychiatric Medications,* coauthored with David Cohen.

Hopefully our work together will illustrate the need for a well-functioning brain and mind that can tap into feelings and make rational choices. However, in recent years most people come to me because they know my views on drugs in advance and they specifically don't want to start them or they want help in stopping them.

Unfortunately, if a patient has been taking drugs for many years, especially neuroleptic or antipsychotic drugs, it can become impossible to stop them. The withdrawal becomes too painful and hazardous, especially outside a hospital.

A Few Words for Therapists

Your Drug May Be Your Problem, written by me and David Cohen, can be useful to professionals who have been propagandized to believe that they must prescribe psychiatric drugs or refer patients to doctors who can do so. Too many therapists who don't believe in drugs nonetheless feel intimidated into referring patients for them. As it turns out, there are very few lawsuits against therapists for not encouraging or participating in drug treatment. By contrast, psychiatrists and other medical doctors are commonly sued for negligence in regard to prescribing drugs.

Therapists who adequately inform their patients about the various treatment alternatives available within the profession, including drugs, and who develop a respectful relationship with their patients, will seldom risk a malpractice lawsuit when they do not choose to refer their patients for drugs. However, these are complex legal and therapeutic issues that cannot be fully addressed in a book that is intended for the general public.

The Importance of
Limiting the Therapy Relationship

Although an empathic, caring relationship lies at the heart of being helpful, professional therapy requires more. First and foremost, it requires a carefully circumscribed or limited relationship.

Only then can the patient feel safe enough to risk entering into a caring relationship. Therefore, personal contact should be carefully limited outside of therapy sessions. So even if your patient is the best accountant in town, or even if you think your therapist would make a wonderful friend, patients and therapists should avoid close contact with each other outside of therapy. Because of human frailty—including the therapist's frailty—therapy as an intense, intimate relationship cannot remain safe if the people are also relating outside the confines of treatment.

Love Is Not Enough

Although the protected, empathic relationship is the core of therapy, many other healing activities usually need to take place. In my own therapy practice, I work hard to help my patients learn more about experiencing their own feelings and about identifying the thinking patterns that guide their behavior. In other words, I try to help them become more aware of the patterns of their feelings and thoughts.

I also help my patients identify past experiences in childhood and adulthood that have discouraged them or led them into self-defeating patterns of relating. The most disabling self-defeating, helpless thoughts and feelings can usually be traced back to lessons learned during childhood. That's because we were truly helpless in childhood, and vulnerable to developing emotional helplessness in the form of depression later in life.

For example, after being rejected by a withdrawn mother and by his first serious girlfriend, a young man may give up seeking love, and lapse into lifelong feelings of sadness and emptiness. Similarly, a woman who was emotionally or physically abused by her alcoholic father and by her first husband may decide that it's impossible to have a safe, loving relationship with a man, and instead remain in a depressing marriage for the rest of her life. People can have difficulty coming to grips with these painful experiences and these self-defeating patterns without the help of therapy.

198 / The Antidepressant Fact Book

I work especially hard trying to help my patients identify the kinds of mistaken lessons they have drawn from childhood, especially the repetitive self-defeating approaches that they have taken in their love, family, and work life. Most people have self-defeating ways of dealing with other people, and sometimes these patterns drive away the people they love or value. They have some awareness of failing in their personal lives, but lack a clear understanding of what they have done to contribute to or to cause these failures.

Unlike many other therapists, I also communicate my values to my patients, especially my emphasis on the creation of noncoercive, mutually respectful, loving relationships everywhere in our lives, including with our spouses, children, coworkers, and friends. I offer my own definition of love as *joyful awareness* of another person or some other aspect of life, and I explain that this kind of joyful awareness tends to lead toward bonding, treasuring, and even reverence.

Many people grow shy and fearful about presenting themselves in a loving way to other people. They need to understand that a loving person does not give up emotional or physical self-defense. Instead, the more loving we become, the more able we become to spot unloving, hostile attitudes that other people may display toward us and our loved ones. As a result, when we are more in touch with our loving nature, we are also more able to identify and to ward off any hostility that is directed toward us.

The Importance of Relationship

People vary a great deal in the importance they place on intimacy with another human being, but in my personal and professional experience, loving intimacy is central to living a satisfying and happy life. For myself, nothing and no one matters as much to me as my wife Ginger, with whom I share every aspect of life. We work and play together all day long, and she is a constant inspiration and source of joy to me.

Too many therapists teach their patients and clients "not to base their happiness on other people." It is necessary to learn to survive without love and intimacy, but it is by no means an ideal way of life. To the contrary, I cannot imagine happiness without ethical, rational, loving people in my life.

The Challenge of Being an Ethical Person and Therapist

In some ways it is more difficult, but in the long run it is far more rewarding to base therapy on the principles I advocate. Many psychiatrists and therapists complain about "burnout." As the years have grown into decades, I have never felt bored, worn out, or otherwise overwhelmed by my private practice of psychiatry. To the contrary, the daily experience of building caring, empathic relationships with other people is revitalizing. To me, it is a blessing to get to know so many people so well, and to help many of them live better lives. I feel grateful to be a psychiatrist and a therapist. As I described in the *Heart of Being Helpful* (1997), the grateful therapist is the best therapist.

By contrast, I have often felt discouraged by my reform efforts. Even when they are immensely successful as they have been at times, a part of me wishes I were devoting less time to active political and professional conflict and confrontation and more time to writing and to therapy. It's worth mentioning this because I do not believe that life is simply a matter of chasing pleasure or even happiness. The satisfaction of living a principled life—a life that meets our ideals—is more to be valued than living a "happy" life. In fact, we cannot readily control how happy our lives will be because happiness in part depends on circumstances, such as our own health and the health of our loved ones, and such as living in a relatively free country versus living under a brutal dictatorship. Living by sound ethical principles makes us less vulnerable to depression and to other helpless feelings, but principled living should be sought for its own sake.

Depression to a great extent is a loss of meaning—a feeling that nothing matters or can matter, a feeling that it's futile to try to make anything matter. Principled living is the ultimate antidote to that feeling. If you decide that you should not, as a human being, waste your life or the life of anyone else, you will find there's always plenty to do that's worthwhile. Your problem, like mine, will be finding the time and energy to deal with all the wonderful challenges and opportunities that life presents.

Doctors Who Practice
Drug-Free Therapy

Many psychiatrists and therapists share my views, although fewer are willing to go through the professional conflict involved in taking public stands as I have done. Dozens of these psychiatrists and therapists belong to the International Center for the Study of Psychiatry and Psychology (see Appendix A). You can hear them speak and meet them at the center's conferences and read their views in the center's journal. But the truth cannot be determined by counting heads. I believe that these principles are most consistent with the Hippocratic oath, which states "First, do no harm." By not locking up people against their will and by not prescribing mind-altering drugs, I do my best to do no harm, and instead try to empower people to think rationally and independently, and to relate to others and to life with their own unique combination of passion and rationality.

Appendix A

International Center for the Study of
Psychiatry and Psychology (ICSPP)
4628 Chestnut Street
Bethesda, MD 20814
301 652-5580

ICSPP is a reform-oriented international center for professionals concerned about ethical and scientific issues in human research and services. It is the only professional organization that has taken a firm public and professional stand against the massive psychiatric drugging of America's children. However, it focuses on the entire field of mental health, including the biological and social sciences.

The board of directors, advisory council, and membership include hundreds of professionals in many fields spanning psychology, counseling, social work, psychiatry, and other medical specialties, neuroscience, education, religion, and law. Former members of the U.S. Congress and other community leaders also belong.

Founded in 1971 by its director, Peter R. Breggin, M.D., ICSPP began its successful reform efforts with opposition to the international resurgence of psychosurgery. In the mid-1990s, ICSPP organized a campaign that caused the U.S. government to withdraw its "violence initiative," a proposed government-wide program that called for intrusive biomedical experiments on inner-city children in the hope of demonstrating biological and genetic causes of violence. ICSPP's most recent reform efforts are directed at the growing trend to psychiatrically diagnose and medicate children.

Because of its many successful efforts on behalf of truthfulness and justice in the psychosocial and biomedical sciences, ICSPP has been called "the conscience of psychiatry."

ICSPP offers a general membership. It publishes a newsletter and periodically distributes news releases and press packages about contemporary issues in the human sciences. Every year or two ICSPP hosts international conferences open to the public and to professionals.

In 1999, ICSPP began its peer-reviewed journal, *Ethical Human Sciences and Services: An International Journal of Critical Inquiry,* published by Springer Publishing Company. In keeping with ICSPP's goals, the journal gives priority to scientific papers and reviews that raise the level of ethical awareness concerning research, theory, and practice.

ICSPP general memberships are $25 (U.S.) in the United States and $35 (U.S.) internationally. Members receive the newsletter, a discount on the journal, and announcements of activities, including meetings.

Further information about ICSPP membership and activities can be obtained on its web sites at www.icspp.org and at www.breggin.com.

Appendix B

Ethical Human Sciences and Services: An International Journal of Critical Inquiry

The mandate of *Ethical Human Sciences and Services: An International Journal of Critical Inquiry (EHSS)* is to understand and address the genuine needs of human beings in an ethical and scientific manner.

EHSS publishes scientific research, literature reviews, clinical reports, commentary, and book reviews that draw on broad ethical and scientific perspectives, including critiques of reductionist theories and practices in various schools of thought and ideology. It spans the fields of psychology, counseling, social work, nursing, sociology, education, public advocacy, public health, and the law, as well as medical fields such as psychiatry, pediatrics, and neurology, and biomedical sciences such as genetics and psychopharmacology.

This peer-review journal seeks to raise the level of scientific knowledge and ethical discourse, at the same time empowering professionals who are devoted to principled human sciences and services unsullied by professional and economic interests.

The coeditors are psychiatrist Peter R. Breggin, M.D., and professor of social work David Cohen, Ph.D. *EHSS* is the official journal of the International Center for the Study of Psychiatry and Psychology. On the editorial advisory board are more than fifty international ICSPP members, including Fred Bemak, Ed.D.;

Phyllis Chesler, Ph.D.; Graham Dukes, M.D., LLD; Alberto Ferguson, M.D.; Giovanni de Girolamo, M.D.; James Gordon, M.D.; Thomas Greening, Ph.D.; Richard Horobin, Ph.D.; Lucy Johnstone, Dip. Clin. Psych.; Bertram Karon, Ph.D.; Kate Millett, Ph.D.; Loren Mosher, M.D.; Dorothy Rowe, Ph.D.; Thomas Scheff, Ph.D.; Clemmont Vontress, Ph.D.; Lenore Walker, Ed.D.; and Wolf Wolfensberger, Ph.D.

The journal welcomes the submission of unsolicited manuscripts. Please send manuscripts and direct editorial inquiries to the editorial office: David Cohen, Ph.D., School of Social Work, Florida International University, University Park, ECS 460, Miami, Florida 33199. Office phone: 305 348-5880. Fax: 305 348-5313. E-mail: cohenda@flu.edu.

Domestic subscription rates are $44 individual and $88 institutional. Outside the United States, rates are $52 (U.S.) individual and $100 (U.S.) institutional. To order a subscription, contact Springer Publishing Company, 536 Broadway, New York, NY 10012-9904. Telephone: 212 431-4370; fax: 212 941-7842.

Notes

Introduction

1. Data from Garnett (May 7, 2000).

2. I have described and documented the power of drug companies to influence research, the government, medical societies, insurance companies, and other institutions of society in several books, including *Toxic Psychiatry* (1991), *Talking Back to Prozac* (with Ginger Breggin, 1994), *Brain-Disabling Treatments in Psychiatry* (1997a), *Talking Back to Ritalin* (1998, rev. ed. 2001), and *The War Against Children of Color* (with Ginger Breggin, 1998). The theme will also be documented throughout this book.

Chapter 1

1. Breggin (1999a, 1999b, and 1999c); Breggin (2001).

Chapter 2

1. Ecstasy is MDMA (methylenedioxymethamphetamine). It has been used extensively since the 1980s as a "recreational" drug. It is known to cause degeneration of serotonin nerve cells and axons in rats (Ricuarte, Byran, Strauss, Seiden, and Schuster, 1985).

2. Klam (January 21, 2001).

3. Freud's self-described love affair with cocaine is documented by his own letters. See Byck (1974).

4. Tardive dyskinesia studies are cited and reviewed in Breggin (1997) and mentioned in Chapter 4 of this book as well.

5. Food and Drug Administration (1997).

6. For a review of fenfluramine-induced primary pulmonary hypertension and neurotoxicity, see McCann et al. (1997). The literature is vast.

7. The neurochemistry I am describing can be confirmed in any textbook of neurochemistry and in many psychiatric textbooks as well. For the scientific research see, for example, Wong et al., (1985) and de Montigny et al. (1990). I review numerous scientific studies in Breggin and Breggin (1994) chap. 7.

8. See Wamsley et al., (1987). See additional references in Breggin and Breggin (1994) chap. 7.

9. Wegerer et al. (1999).

10. Bergqvist et al. (1999).

11. Gilbert et al. (2000). To evade facing the damage caused by Paxil, the authors speculate that the children had abnormally large thalami and that the drug may have corrected this by shrinking their brains.

12. Malberg et al., 2000. See Weaver (2000) for the press release from Yale University.

13. Freo et al. (2000).

14. Norrholm and Ouimet (November 2000). The specific abnormality was an increase in dendritic length and spine density.

15. Kalia et al. (2000).

16. Fuller, 1994 (266).

Chapter 3

1. The material about stimulation in this chapter is documented with dozens of citations to the literature and to FDA and drug company documents in Breggin and Breggin (1994) and in Breggin (1997a). In this chapter, I focus more specifically on data found in the label of the drug (*Physicians' Desk Reference*, 2001) because it is readily available to the reader in most libraries.

2. American Psychiatric Association (1994), 331.

3. Emsley et al. (1999), 1033, for passing mention of children developing manic symptoms on Prozac in the clinical trials.

4. Kapit (October 17, 1986), 18, for data on Prozac-induced mania.

5. Zwillich (June 2000). The quote is the reporter's paraphrasing.

6. *Physicians' Desk Reference* (2001). The adverse drug effects with a range of percentages are taken from table 1 and table 2 on page 1130 and the adverse drug effects labeled "frequent" are taken from the "Nervous System" category in the third column on the same page.

7. Lipinski et al. (1989) and Rothschild and Locke (1991) describe SSRI-induced akathisia. Van Putten (1975) describes generic akathisia caused by neuroleptics.

Chapter 4

1. For a review see *Drug Facts and Comparisons* (2001, 930ff).

2. Leo (1996).

3. See Breggin (1997) for detailed documentation about tardive dyskinesia caused by neuroleptics.

4. For details of the case, see www.breggin.com.

5. I document the rates with many citations to the literature in Breggin (1997a). Also see Breggin and Cohen (1999).

6. Budman and Bruun (1991).

7. Sandler (1996).

8. *Drug Facts and Comparisons* (2001), 931.

9. Ibid.

10. Chambers et al. (1996).

11. The word "completely" is from a letter by Johns (2000). Although serotonin neurons do not connected directly to these glandular cells, Prozac seemed to affect the cells by a

mechanism similar to its impact on nerve cells. Prozac blocked the ability of the gland cells to take up serotonin.

Chapter 5

1. Patterson (1993).

Chapter 6

1. Kapit (March 1986).

2. Reviewed in Breggin (1997) 92–94.

3. Health Letter (June 1990).

4. American Psychiatric Association (1994), 331. Although the manual seldom comments on adverse drug effects, it mentions antidepressant-induced mania and mood disorders several times.

5. Cherland and Fitzpatrick (1999). The authors believe the true rates of Ritalin-induced psychosis were even higher than reported in the records.

6. Frankenfield et al. (1994).

7. Moore, T. (December 1997). Hard to swallow. *The Washingtonian*, 69ff.

8. See Chapter 3.

9. American Psychiatric Association (1994), 745.

10. Glenmullen's (2000) scientific analysis of how SSRIs can cause suicide, violence, and other behavioral aberrations is essentially the same as my earlier detailed analyses (Breggin and Breggin, 1994; Breggin, 1997), my hundreds of media appearances, and my testimony in court cases that Glenmullen also had available. Glenmullen also interviewed my wife and coauthor Ginger Breggin for his book and was sent research documents from our files that he was otherwise unable to obtain. Disappointingly, in his book Glenmullen literally expurgates our contribution, never mentioning my origination of the ideas he was espousing and never acknowledging my efforts as the primary critic of SSRIs in the scientific and legal arena. Glenmullen made it sound as if he'd thought it up all on his own. Nonetheless, his book provides a service in updating limited aspects of my earlier books with more recent clinical and research publications.

11. The California attorneys in the case are Vince Nguyen and Don Farber.

12. Reboxetine, not available in the United States, is a selective noradrenaline reuptake inhibitor.

13. These and other studies of SSRI-induced suicidality are discussed in Breggin (1997a).

14. Petersen (August 10, 2000), Appleby (August 10, 2000), and Reuters (August 9, 2000).

15. For a discussion of the "new Prozac," see Garnett (May 7, 2000). The quotes around new and old Prozac are mine.

Chapter 7

1. The case is *State of Connecticut vs. DeAngelo* (February 2000).

2. See my chapter on benzodiazepines in my 1997 textbook, *Brain-Disabling Treatments in Psychiatry,* or my scientific report on the same subject published in 1998.

3. Some of these "Prozac defense" cases are described on my web site: www.breggin.com. Also see Breggin and Breggin (1994).

4. American Psychiatric Association (1994, 328–330).

5. I discussed the FDA's study of Prozac and violence in my 1994 testimony in the Wesbecker case and in my book *Brain-Disabling Treatments in Psychiatry* (1997). Other than the original documents, there is no other source for the information.

Chapter 8

1. MAOI stands for monoamine oxidase inhibitors.

2. DeVane (1988, 164 ff.) provides a good general description of the array of liver enzymes that affect drug metabolism. A number can be genetically weaker or absent.

3. Sallee et al. (2000).

Chapter 9

1. Zito et al. (2000) and for a commentary, Coyle (2000).

2. Wegerer et al. (1999). The Prozac dose given in the water was 5mg/kg/per day. The brain changes persisted ninety days later in the now adult rats. In Chapter 2, I discussed SSRI-induced loss of receptors (downregulation). In this study, the Prozac caused an increase in the transporter system, which would have increased the removal rate of serotonin from the synapse. This, like downregulation of the receptors, would have the overall effect of compensating for overstimulation by the drug, since Prozac would be removed more readily by the increased number of transporters.

3. Gilbert et al. (1990). The reduced brain volume was in the thalamus. The children were ages eight to seventeen. The study claims that the OCD children originally had larger thalami and that the drugs then decreased the volume. The alleged increased size of the thalami in OCD children is unlikely, and reflects a complex assessment involving a control group for comparison. But the shrinkage is a more definitive fact as it was measured with before-and-after brain scans in the same children during the time the children were under treatment with Paxil.

4. Riddle et al. (1990–1991).

5. Jain et al. (1992).

6. Emslie et al. (1997).

7. Breggin (September 1995).

8. For a further analysis of Eric Harris's use of Luvox, see Breggin, (2000a).

9. Information from the *Physicians' Desk Reference* (2001), section on Luvox.

10. Wilkinson cites Hoehn-Saric et al. (1990) concerning SSRI-induced apathy, indifference, or blunting.

11. American Psychiatric Association (1999).

12. Fred is my name for him. He was called "F."

13. Baker (1995).

14. Sommers-Flanagan and Sommers-Flanagan (1996).

Chapter 10

1. Discussed in Breggin (1997a) and in Breggin and Cohen (1999).

2. A detailed review of antidepressant withdrawal reactions and more detailed suggestions on how to withdraw from psychiatric drugs can be found in Breggin and Cohen (1999).

3. Schatzberg et al. (1997b), 4–5.

4. Haddad (1997), 21.

Chapter 11

1. Scientific studies confirming the role of environmental factors in emotional suffering are reviewed in my books *Beyond Conflict* (1992), *Reclaiming Our Children* (2000) and *Talking Back to Ritalin* (1998, revised in 2001).

2. Blumenthal et al. (1999) showed that exercise was as effective as Zoloft after sixteen weeks of treatment and Babyak et al. (2000) showed that exercise was more effective than Zoloft after ten months.

Chapter 12

1. Bower, B. "Placebos for Depression Attract Scrutiny." *Science News 157* (April 29, 2000): 278.

2. The information reviewed in this section is documented in sources such as Greenberg and Greenberg (1989, 1995, 1997), Kirsch and Sapirstein (1998), and Antonuccio et al. (1994, 1995). It is also discussed in Breggin (1991, 1997a).

3. For Ritalin class act information see www.breggin.com and www.Ritalinfraud.com.

4. These documents are described and quoted in Breggin (1997a), 228–230.

5. For a variety of studies concerning the relative effects of antidepressants and placebo, see Fisher and Greenberg (1989, 1995, and 1997). For more about the limits of the FDA approval process, see Breggin (1997a).

Chapter 13

1. See Blumenthal et al. (1999), Babyak et al. (2000) and discussion at end of chapter.

2. I describe the brain-disabling principle of treatment in psychiatry in greatest detail in my 1997 medical book, *Brain-Disabling Treatments in Psychiatry*.

3. Rodgers (1992), 209. I have written about the antipsychosurgery campaign in greatest detail in chapter 6 in *The War Against Children of Color* (1998, with Ginger Breggin). The chapter provides many citations to the literature and to my other writings on the subject of psychosurgery.

4. Borzo (November 2000).

5. Thomas R. was also described in their publications as Leonard K, his real name. I tell his story with detailed scientific documentation in *The War Against Children of Color* (1994).

6. The study is Kroessler and Fogel (1993). Burke et al. (1987) describe some of the complications among the elderly. See Breggin (1997a) for other citations.

7. Bratman and Kroll (1999).

8. Breggin (1979, 1991, 1997a, 1998b).

9. Sackeim et al. (1993).

10. Wirth (1991). This information was taken from a deposition under oath given by Dr. Wirth when he was on the staff of Johns Hopkins.

Chapter 14

1. Bratman and Krol (1998) have a lengthy section devoted to herbs for depression, including summaries of adverse effects. The authors mention that St. John's wort increases P450 enzyme activity. Ironically, they carefully scrutinize claims for safety and efficacy of herbs but they promote the drug company line when it comes to FDA-approved antidepressants. For example, they claim that FDA-approved antidepressants are more effective in severe depression and in suicide, when there is no scientific evidence for the claim. The *PDR for Herbal Medicines* (1998) covers most available substances. Maleskey's (1999) *Nature's Medicines* provides interesting background information. Brinker's (1998) *Herb Contraindications and Drug Interactions* is somewhat incomplete but useful for professionals and laypersons alike.

2. See note 1 for some relevant books.

Chapter 15

1. *Not* the psychiatrist Lee Coleman of California.

2. Data on suicide, violence, agitation, akathisia, and mania caused by Prozac are discussed in Chapters 6 and 7 of this book, and in more detail in Breggin and Breggin (1994) and Breggin (1997a).

3. Castellanos (1995) Potter (1995); Scanlon (1995), and most extensively, Varchaver (1995).

4. Varchaver (1995).

5. My letter is Breggin (1992b) and the American Psychiatric Association's rebuttal letter is Sabshin (1992).

Bibliography

American Psychiatric Association. *Diagnostic and Statistical Manual of Mental Disorders,* vol. 4. Washington, D.C.: American Psychiatric Association (1994).

Antonuccio, D. O., W. G. Danton, and G. Y. DeNelsky. "Psychotherapy: No Stronger Medicine." *Scientist Practitioner* 4, no. 1 (1994): 2–18.

_____. "Psychotherapy Versus Medication for Depression: Challenging the Conventional Wisdom with Data." *Professional Psychology: Research and Practice* 26 (1995): 574–585.

Appleby, J. "Eli Lilly Loses Fight for Prozac." *USA Today* (August 10, 2000): 1B.

Babyak, M., J. Blumenthal, S. Herman, P. Khatri, M. Doraiswamy, K. Moore, W. Craighead, T. Baldewicz, and K. Krishnan. "Exercise Treatment for Major Depression." *Psychosomatic Medicine* 62 (2000): 633.

Bauer, B. "Placebos for Depression Attract Scrutiny." *Science News* 157 (April 29, 2000): 278.

Bergqvist, P., C. Bouchard, and P. Blier. "Effect of Long-Term Administration of Antidepressant Treatments on Serotonin Release in the Brain Regions Involved in Obsessive-Compulsive Disorder." *Biological Psychiatry* 45 (1999): 164–174.

Blumenthal, J., M. Babyak, K. Moore, W. Craighead, S. Herman, P. Khatri, R. Waugh, M. Napolitano, L. Forman, M. Appelbaum, P. Doraiswamy, and K. Krishnan. "Effects of Exercise Training on Older Patients with Major Depression." *Archives of Internal Medicine* 159 (1999): 2349–2356.

Bodenheimer, T. "Uneasy Alliance: Clinical Investigators and the Pharmaceutical Industry." *New England Journal of Medicine* 324 (May 18, 2000): 1539–1544.

Borenstein, D. "Pharmaceutical Companies." *Psychiatric News* (November 17, 2000): 3.

Borzo, G. "Brain Stimulation for Refractory Mood Disorders? Still Experimental." *Clinical Psychiatry News* (November 2000): 26.

Bower (2000). Bower, B. "Placebos for Depression Attract Scrutiny." *Science News 157* (April 29, 2000): 278.

Bratman, S., and D. Kroll. *Natural Health Bible*. www.thenaturalpharma-cist.com: Prima Health, 1999.

Breggin, P. "Brain Damage, Dementia and Persistent Cognitive Dysfunction Associated with Neuroleptic Drugs: Evidence, Etiology, Implications." *Journal of Mind and Behavior* 11 (1990): 425–464.

_____. *Toxic Psychiatry: Why Therapy, Empathy and Love Must Replace the Drugs, Electroshock and Biochemical Theories of the "New Psychiatry."* New York: St. Martin's Press, 1991.

_____. *Beyond Conflict: From Self-Help and Psychotherapy to Peacemaking*. New York: St. Martin's Press, 1992a.

_____. "The President's Sleeping Pill and Its Makers" (letter). *New York Times* (February 11, 1992b): A18.

_____. "A Case of Fluoxetine-Induced Stimulant Side Effects with Suicidal Ideation Associated with a Possible Withdrawal Reaction ('Crashing')." *International Journal of Risk and Safety in Medicine* 3 (1992c): 325–328.

_____. "Parallels Between Neuroleptic Effects and Lethargic Encephalitis: The Production of Dyskinesias and Cognitive Disorders." *Brain and Cognition* 23 (1993): 8–27.

_____. "Prozac 'Hazardous' to Children" (letter). *Clinical Psychiatry News* (September 1995): 10.

_____. *Brain-Disabling Treatments in Psychiatry: Drugs, Electroshock and the Role of the FDA*. New York: Springer Publishing Company, 1997a.

_____. *The Heart of Being Helpful: Empathy and the Creation of a Healing Presence*. New York: Springer Publishing Company, 1997b.

_____. "Psychotherapy in Emotional Crises Without Resort to Psychiatric Medication." *Humanistic Psychologist* 25 (1997c): 2–14.

_____. "Analysis of Adverse Behavioral Effects of Benzodiazepines with a Discussion on Drawing Scientific Conclusions from the FDA's spontaneous Reporting System." *Journal of Mind and Behavior* 19 (1998a): 21–50.

_____. "Electroshock: Scientific, Ethical, and Political Issues." *International Journal of Risk and Safety in Medicine* 11 (1998b): 5-40.

_____. "Risks and Mechanism of Action of Stimulants." *Program and Abstracts* (November 16–18, 1998c): 105–120. NIH Consensus Development Conference on the Diagnosis and Treatment of Attention Deficit Hyperactivity Disorder. William H. Natcher Conference Center. National Institutes of Health. Bethesda, Maryland.

_____. "Psychostimulants in the Treatment of Children Diagnosed with ADHD: Part I: Acute Risks and Psychological Effects." *Ethical Human Sciences and Services* 1 (1999a): 13–33.

_____. "Psychostimulants in the Treatment of Children Diagnosed with ADHD: Part II: Adverse Effects on Brain and Behavior." *Ethical Human Sciences and Services* 1 (1999b): 213–241.

_____. "Psychostimulants in the Treatment of Children Diagnosed with ADHD: Risks and Mechanism of Action. *International Journal of Risk and Safety in Medicine* 12 (1999c): 3–35. By special arrangement, this report was originally published in two parts by Springer Publishing Company in *Ethical Human Sciences and Services* (Breggin 1999a, 1999b).

_____. *Reclaiming Our Children: A Healing Solution for a Nation in Crisis*. Cambridge, Mass.: Perseus Books, 2000a.

_____. "Don't Let 'Experts' Parent Your Children." *USA Today* (February 28, 2000b): 19A.

_____. "What Psychologists and Psychotherapists Need to Know About ADHD and Stimulants." *Changes: An International Journal of Psychology and Psychotherapy* 18 (spring 2000c): 13–23.

_____. September 29, 2000d. Testimony concerning behavioral drug use in the schools before the U.S. House of Representatives Committee on Education and the Workforce, Subcommittee on Oversight and Investigations, Washington, D.C. Text of Breggin's formal submission to the committee available at www.breggin.com. See U.S. House of Representatives, 2000, for how to purchase C-Span film of entire hearing.

_____. *Talking Back to Ritalin: What Doctors Aren't Telling You About Stimulants for Children,* rev. ed. Cambridge, Mass.: Perseus Books, 2001.

Breggin, P., and G. Breggin. *Talking Back to Prozac*. New York: St. Martin's Press, 1994.

_____. *The War Against Children of Color*. Monroe, Maine: Common Courage Press, 1998.

Breggin, P., and D. Cohen. *Your Drug May Be Your Problem: How and Why to Stop Taking Psychiatric Medication*. Cambridge, Mass.: Perseus, 1999.

Breggin, P., and E. M. Stern, eds. *Psychosocial Approaches to Deeply Disturbed Persons*. New York: Haworth Press, 1996.

Brinker, F. *Herb Contraindications and Drug Interactions*. Sandy, Oreg.: Eclectic Medical Publications, 1998.

Budman, C., and Bruun, R. "Persistent Dyskinesia in a Patient Receiving Fluoxetine." *American Journal of Psychiatry* 148 (1991): 1403.

Byck, R., ed. *Cocaine Papers by Sigmund Freud*. New York: New American Library, 1974.

Chambers, C., K. Johnson, L. Dick, R. Felix, and K. Jones. "Birth Outcomes in Pregnant Women Taking Fluoxetine." *New England Journal of Medicine* 335 (1996): 1010–1115.

Cherland, E., and R. Fitzpatrick. "Psychotic Side Effects of Psychostimulants: A 5-Year Review." *Canadian Journal of Psychiatry* 44 (1999): 811–813.

Coyle, J. "Psychotropic Drug Use in Very Young Children." *Journal of the American Medical Association* 283 (February 23, 2000): 1059–1060.

DeVane, C. L. "Principles of Pharmacokinetics and Pharmacodynamics." In *The American Psychiatric Press Textbook of Psychiatry,* edited by A. F. Schatzberg and C. B. Nemeroff, 155–169. Washington, D.C.: American Psychiatric Press, 1998.

Emsley, G., A. Rush, W. Weinberg, R. Kowatch, C. Hughes, T. Carmody, and J. Rinteimann. "A Double-Blind, Randomized, Placebo-Controlled Trial of Fluoxetine in Children and Adolescents with Depression." *Archives of General Psychiatry* 54 (1997): 1031–1037.

Fisher, S., and R. Greenberg, eds. *The Limits of Biological Treatments for Psychological Distress: Comparisons with Psychotherapy and Placebo.* Hillsdale, N.J.: Erlbaum, 1989.

———. "Prescriptions for Happiness." *Psychology Today* (September/October 1995): 32–37.

Fisher, S., and R. Greenberg, eds. *From Placebo to Panacea: Putting Psychiatric Drugs to the Test.* New York: Wiley, 1997.

Food and Drug Administration. "FDA Public Health Advisory Concerning Reports of Valvular Heart Disease in Patients Receiving Concomitant Fenfluramine and Phentermine." *FDA Medical Newsletter* 27, no. 2 (July 8, 1997): 2.

Frankenfield, D., S. Baker, W. Lange, Y. Caplan, and J. Smialek. "Fluoxetine and Violent Death in Maryland." *Forensic Science International* 64 (1964): 107–111.

Freo, U., C. Ori, M. Dam, A. Merico, and G. Pizzolato. "Effects of Acute and Chronic Treatment with Fluoxetine on Regional Glucose Cerebral Metabolism in Rats: Implications for Clinical Therapies." *Brain Research* 854 (2000): 35–41.

Fuller, R. Deposition. Vol. I., in *Fentress et al. v. Shea Communications et al.,* Jefferson Circuit Court, Division One, No. 90-Cl-6033, April 14, 1994.

Garnett, L. R. "Prozac Revisited: A Drug Gets Remade, Concerns About Suicide Surface." *Boston Globe* (May 7, 2000).

Gilbert, A., G. Moore, M. Keshavan, L. Paulson, V. Narula, P. MacMaster, C. Stewart, and D. Rosenberg. "Decreased Thalamic Volumes of Pediatric Patients with Obsessive-Compulsive Disorder Who Are Taking Paroxetine." *Archives of General Psychiatry* 57 (2000): 449–456.

Glenmullen, J. *Prozac Backlash.* New York: Simon and Schuster, 2000.

Healy, D. *The Antidepressant Era.* Cambridge, Mass.: Harvard University Press, 1997.

———. "Reply to D. Wilkinson—Loss of Anxiety and Increased Aggression in a 15-Year-Old Boy Taking Fluoxetine." *Journal of Psychopharmacology* 13 (1999): 421.

———. "Emergence of Antidepressant Induced Suicidality." *Primary Care Physician* 6 (2000): 23–28.

Healy, D., C. Langmaack, and M. Savage, M. "Suicides in the Course of the Treatment of Depression." *Journal of Psychopharmacology* 13 (1999): 94–99.

Hoehn-Saric, R., J. Lipsey, and D. McLeod. "Apathy and Indifference in Patients on Fluvoxamine and Fluoxetine." *Journal of Clinical Psychopharmacology* 10 (1990): 343–345.

Jain, J., B. Birmaher, M. Garcia, M. Al-Shabbout, and N. Ryan. "Fluoxetine in Children and Adolescents with Mood Disorders: A Chart Review of Efficacy and Adverse Reactions." *Journal of Child and Adolescent Psychopharmacology* 2 (1992): 259–265.

Johns, M. Letter to the *New York Times*, unpublished (July 27, 2000).

Johns, M., E. Azmitia, and D. Krieger. "Specific In Vitro Uptake of Serotonin in the Anterior Pituitary of the Rat." *Endocrinology* 110 (1982): 754–760.

Johns, M., E. C. Azmitia, E. A. Zimmerman, and D. T. Krieger. "Specific *In Vitro* Uptake of [^{3}H]-5HT in the Pituitary of the Rat." *Society of Neuroscience Abstracts* 6 (1980): 855.

Kalia, M., J. O'Callaghan, D. Miller, and M. Kramer. "Comparative Study of Fluoxetine, Sibutramine, Sertraline and Dexfenfluramine on the Morphology of Serotonergic Nerve Terminals Using Serotonin Immunohistochemistry." *Brain Research* 858 (2000): 92–105.

Kapit, R. "Safety Update. New Drug Application (NDA-18-936)." Internal document of the Department of Health and Human Services, Public Health Service, Food and Drug Administration, Center for Drug Evaluation and Research. Obtained through the Freedom of Information Act. October 17, 1986.

King, Robert A., Mark A. Riddle, Phillip B. Chappell, Maureen T. Hardin, George M. Anderson, Paul Lombroso, and Larry Scahill. "Emergence of Self-Destructive Phenomena in Children and Adolescents During Fluoxetine Treatment." *Journal of the American Academy of Child and Adolescent Psychiatry* 30 (March 1991): 179–186.

Kirsch, I., and G. Sapirstein. "Listening to Prozac but Hearing Placebo: A Meta-Analysis of Antidepressant Medication." *Prevent and Treatment* 1, art. 0002a (June 26, 1998). "http://journals.apa.org.prevention/volume"; http://journals.apa.org.prevention/volume; 1pre0010002a.html.

Klam, M. "Experiencing Ecstasy." *New York Times Magazine* (January 21, 2001): 38ff.

Leo, R. "Movement Disorders Associated with Serotonin Selective Reuptake Inhibitors." *Journal of Clinical Psychiatry* 57 (1996): 449–545.

Lipinksi, J., Jr., G. Mallaya, P. Zimmerman, and G. Pope Jr. "Fluoxetine-Induced Akathisia: Clinical and Theoretical Implications." *Journal of Clinical Psychiatry* 50 (September 1989): 339–342.

Malberg, J., A. Eisch, E. Nestler, and R. Duman. "Chronic Antidepressant Treatment Increases Neurogenesis in Adult Rat Hippocampus." *Journal of Neuroscience* 20 (December 15, 2000): 9104–9110.

Maleskey, G. *Nature's Medicines.* Emmaus, Pa.: Rodale Press, 1999.

McCann, U., L. Seiden, L. Rubin, and A. Ricuarte. "Brain Serotonin Neurotoxicity and Primary Pulmonary Hypertension from Fenfluramine and Dexfenfluramine: A Systematic Review of the Evidence." *Journal of the American Medical Association* 278 (August 27, 1997): 666–672.

Medical Letter. "Some Drugs That Cause Psychiatric Symptoms." *The Medical Letter* 40, no. 1020 (February 13, 1998).

Montigny, C. de, I. Chaput, and P. Blier. "Modification of Serotonergic Neuron Properties by Long-Term Treatment with Serotonin Reuptake Blockers." *Journal of Clinical Psychiatry* 51, supp. B (December 1990): 12.

Moore, T. "Hard to Swallow." *Washingtonian* (December 1997): 69 ff.

Mynors-Wallis, L., D. Gath, A. Day, and F. Baker. "Randomized Controlled Trial of Problem Solving Treatment, Antidepressant Medication, and Combined Treatment for Major Depression in Primary Care." *General Practice* 320 (2000): 26–30.

Norrholm, S., and C. Ouimet. "Chronic Fluoxetine Administration to Juvenile Rats Prevents Age-Associated Dendritic Proliferation in Hippocampus." *Brain Research* 883 (2000): 205–215.

Patterson, William. "Fluoxetine-Induced Sexual Dysfunction." *Journal of Clinical Psychiatry* 54 (February 1993): 71.

PDR for Herbal Medicines. Montvale, N.J.: Medical Economics, 1998.

Petersen, M. "Lilly Setback in Patient Case over Prozac." *New York Times* (August 10, 2000): C1.

Physicians' Desk Reference. Montvale, N.J.: Medical Economics, 2001.

Public Citizen Health Research Group. "Health Letter: Drug-Induced Depression." Washington, D.C.: Public Citizen Health Research Group, June 1990.

Putten, T. van, "The Many Faces of Akathisia." Comprehensive Psychiatry 16 (1975b): 43–47.

Reuters. "Lilly Setback by Court Ruling on Prozac." Reuters (August 9, 2000).

Ricuarte, G., G. Byran, L. Strauss, L. Seiden, and C. Schuster. "Hallucinogenic Amphetamine Selectively Destroys Brain Serotonin Nerve Terminals." *Science* 229 (1985): 986–988.

Riddle, Mark A., Robert A. King, Maureen T. Hardin, Lawrence Scahill, Sharon Ort, Phillip Chappell, Ann Rasmusson, and James F. Leckman. "Behavioral Side of Fluoxetine in Children and Adolescents." *Journal of Child and Adolescent Psychopharmacology* 1 (1990/1991): 193–198.

Rothschild, A., and C. Locke. "Reexposure to Fluoxetine: After Serious Suicide Attempts by Three Patients: The Role of Akathisia." *Journal of Clinical Psychiatry* 52 (1991): 491–493.

Rustad, M. "Antidepressants Found to Alter Brain Cells in Rats. *Medical Tribune* (July 3, 2000): www.medtrib.com.

Rybacki, J., and J. Long. *The Essential Guide to Prescription Drugs.* New York: HarperCollins, 2000.

Sabshin, M. "To Aid Understanding of Mental Disorders" (letter). *New York Times* (March 10, 1992): A24.

Sallee, F. R., C. L. DeVane, and R. E. Ferrell. "Fluoxetine-Related Death in a Child with Cytochrome P450 2D6 Genetic Deficiency." *Journal of Child and Adolescent Psychopharmacology* 10 (2000): 27–34.

Sandler, N. "Tardive Dyskinesia Associated with Fluoxetine." *Journal of Clinical Psychiatry* 57 (1996): 91.

Teicher, M. H., C. A. Glod, and J. O. Cole. "Emergence of Intense Suicidal Preoccupations During Fluoxetine Treatment." *American Journal of Psychiatry* 147 (February 1990): 207–210.

_____. "Antidepressant Drugs and the Emergence of Suicidal Tendencies." *Drug Safety* 8, no. 3 (1993): 186–212.

Walker, P., J. Cole, E. Gardner, A. Hughes, A. Johnson, S. Batey, and C. Lineberry. "Improvement in Fluoxetine-Associated Sexual Dysfunction in Patients Switched to Buproprion." *Journal of Clinical Psychiatry* 54 (1993): 459–465.

Wamsley, J. K., W. F. Byerley, R. T. McCabe, E. J. McConnell, T. M. Dawson, and B. I. Grosser. "Receptor Alterations Associated with Serotonergic Agents: An Autographic Analysis." *Journal of Clinical Psychiatry* 48, no. 3 (supp, 1987): 19–85.

Weaver, J. "Sustained Use of Anti-Depressants Increases Cell Growth and Protects Cells in the Brain" (press release). New Haven, Conn.: Yale University, December 15, 2000.

Wegerer, V., G. Moll, M. Bagli, A. Rothenberger, E. Ruther, and G. Huether. "Persistently Increased Density of Serotonin Transporters in the Frontal Cortex of Rats Treated with Fluoxetine During Early Juvenile Life." *Journal of Child and Adolescent Psychopharmacology* 9 (1999): 13–24.

Wilkinson, D. "Loss of Anxiety and Increased Aggression in a 15-Year-Old Taking Fluoxetine." *Journal of Psychopharmacology* 13 (1999): 420–421.

Wong, D., L. Reid, F. Bymaster, and P. Threlkeid. "Chronic Effects of Fluoxetine, a Selective Inhibitor of Serotonin Uptake, on Neurotransmitter Receptors." *Journal of Neural Transmission* 64 (1985): 25-269.

Zito, J., D. Safer, S. dosReis, J. Gardner, M. Boles, and F. Lynch. "Trends in Prescribing Psychotropic Medications to Preschoolers." *Journal of the American Medical Association* 283 (February 23, 2000): 1025–1059.

Zwillich, T. "SSRI Prescribing in Primary Care Draws Fire." *Clinical Psychiatry News* (June 2000): 34.

Index

About the Author

Peter R. Breggin, M.D., is a psychiatrist in full-time private practice in Bethesda, Maryland, where he has treated adults, children, and families since 1968. He gives workshops and frequently appears in the media as an expert on national programs such as *60 Minutes*, *20/20*, and *Nightline*.

Dr. Breggin is one of the world's foremost critics of biological psychiatry, including medication, and is a strong advocate for psychological and social human services. He is the founder and director of the International Center for the Study of Psychiatry and Psychology, a reform-oriented research and educational network. He is also the founder and coeditor of *Ethical Human Sciences and Services*. Dr. Breggin has been on the faculty of the counseling departments of the University of Maryland and Johns Hopkins University, and has also taught at George Mason University and the Washington School of Psychiatry.

Trained at Harvard College and Case Western Reserve Medical School, his three years of residency in psychiatry were at the Massachusetts Mental Health Center, where he was a teaching fellow at Harvard Medical School, and at the State University of New York, Upstate Medical Center. He is a former officer in the U.S. Public Health Service and a former full-time consultant with the National Institute of Mental Health (NIMH).

Dr. Breggin is an editor for several peer review journals. He has published many professional articles and books, including *Toxic Psychiatry* (1991), *Talking Back to Prozac* (1994, with Ginger Breggin), *Brain-Disabling Treatments in Psychiatry* (1997), *The Heart of Being Helpful* (1997), *The War Against Children of Color* (1998, with Ginger Breggin), *Your Drug May Be Your Problem: How and Why to Stop Taking Psychiatric Medication* (1999, with David Cohen), and *Reclaiming Our Children* (2000). A revised edition of *Talking Back to Retalin* (1998) will be published in 2001.

Breggin participates as a medical expert in a variety of forensic activities, including malpractice, criminal, and product liability lawsuits. He was the medical consultant authorized to evaluate the scientific basis for the "combined Prozac suits" against Eli Lilly and Co., the manufacturer of Prozac. Recently his research provided the basis for the current series of class action lawsuits against Novartis, the manufacturer of Ritalin.

More information about Dr. Breggin and his work can be found on his web site, www.breggin.com.